Measuring and Recording

Instrumentation and Techni

John J. Gerhardt
Jules Rippstein

Measuring and Recording of Joint Motion

Instrumentation and Techniques

2nd completely revised and expanded edition of
International SFTR Method of Measuring and Recording
Joint Motion

Medical Illustrations by Marie Valleroy
Graphic Arts by Brian Demings

Hogrefe & Huber Publishers
Toronto · Lewiston, NY · Bern · Göttingen · Stuttgart

Library of Congress Cataloging-in-Publication Data
Gerhardt, John J.
Measuring and recording of joint motion: instrumentation and techniques
John J. Gerhardt and Jules R. Rippstein;
Marie Valleroy (medical illustrator), Brian Demings (graphic artist).
Includes bibliographies.
ISBN 0-920887-33-3
1. Joints — Range of motion – Measurement. 2. Goniometry.
I. Rippstein, Jules R. II. Title.
(DNLM: 1. Joints – physiology. 2. Orthopedic Equipment. WE 300 G368p)
RD734.G475   1990
617'.30028 – dc20
DNLM/DLC

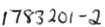

Canadian Cataloguing in Publication Data
Gerhardt, John J.
Measuring and recording of joint motion: instrumentation and techniques
Bibliography: p.
ISBN 0-920887-33-3
1. Joints – Range of motion – Measurement.
I. Rippstein, Jules R. II. Title.
RD734.G47X   1990   617'.3   C90-093949-7

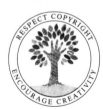

P.O. Box 51
Lewiston, NY 14092

12–14 Bruce Park Avenue
Toronto, Ontario M4P2S3

Printed in Switzerland

ISBN 0-920887-33-3
Hans Huber Publishers, Toronto Lewiston, NY Bern Stuttgart
ISBN 3-456-81805-X
Hans Huber Publishers, Bern · Stuttgart · Toronto · Lewiston, NY

PREFACE

Advantages in science require quantification, and quantification requires accurate measurements. Dr. John Gerhardt designed a measuring and recording system that is a combination of several systems, which he named the SFTR System. Dr. Otto Russe introduced and propagated this method in Europe.

This method allows for precise and easily reproducible measurements of joint ranges of motion. These numeric notations avoid the ambiguity of narrative recording, allowing for great accuracy and brevity.

In investigations of joint functions and the automated analysis of gait accuracy of joint motion, records are essential both for the interpretation of studies and for later comparative analysis of multiple studies. Only by the use of the universal languages of numbers, will we be able to progress in our understanding of the complexities of kinesiology.

Dr. Jules Rippstein facilitated the use of this method and added greatly to the accuracy and almost foolproof reproducibility of measurements by designing his unique Plurimeter precision measuring instrumentation.

The authors deserve our gratitude for developing this simple yet highly accurate method of measuring and recording the range of motion and positions of the joints.

Paul Campbell, M.D.
Clinical Professor of Orthopedic Surgery
Oregon Health Sciences University
Chief of Staff, Shriners Hospital for Crippled Children
Portland, Oregon, U.S.A.

DEDICATED To I.R.M.A.

the International Rehabilition Medicine Association
whose goals are rehabilitation and facilitation of
communication among all medical specialties
internationally.

FOREWORD

Science works through communication. Aggregates of knowledge, even the great singular scientific breakthroughs, are almost never the result of one mind or one intellect. Inevitably then, for progress, scientists must know and understand what other scientists are doing.

The international scientific community has largely eliminated time lag, regional isolation, and language differences as barriers to knowledge interchange. The most formidable obstacles to free communication today are specialization and a lack of standard systems of measurements.

More specialization and fragmentation are unavoidable with the awesome geometric increase of scientific information. International standardization of measurements, concise and workable, can, however, thread a common denominator through the labor of all investigators. Each knows in exact terms what the other is doing. Drs. Gerhardt and Russe here present a practical manual of international standard orthopedic measurements. Their accomplishments in this area are significant and longstanding. The system presented is a meaningful contribution to understanding and data collection in orthopedic surgery and rehabilitation. Its widespread use will simplify and accelerate knowledge accrual. The authors and those associated with them in the preparation of this manual have our gratitude.

Ernest M. Burgess, M.D.
Clinical Professor of Orthopedic Surgery
University of Washington,
School of Medicine,
Seattle, Washington, U.S.A.

ACKNOWLEDGEMENTS

Our gratitude goes to all those who by their work laid the groundwork that eventually led to the development of this method, and to all those who helped propagate it worldwide.

Our thanks go to Professor Ernest Burgess, M.D., for reviewing the original manuscript and writing the foreword and to Professor Paul Campbell, M.D., for writing the preface and for introducing this method for use in gait laboratories.

We would also like to acknowledge the excellent work provided by Mrs. Sara J. Walter in word processing and proofreading the revised manuscript, and to Mr. Wesley E. Schroeder and Mrs. Rosemarie A. Schroeder of Challenger Graphics for assistance in preparing the manuscript and the typesetting of this manual.

Thanks also go to Dr. Marie Valleroy, who drew new illustrations. Her profound medical knowledge combined with her artistry facilitated the success for review of the anatomical and kinesiological considerations, as well as providing the basis for correct application of the measuring instruments. And to Mr. Brian Demings, A.M.I., the graphic artist who provided a clear understanding of measuring and documentation through his explicit artwork.

Last but not least we would like to thank our publisher, Hogrefe & Huber International, for understanding our needs, for their encouragement, and for allowing us to use the larger, more appealing format of the pocketbook.

TABLE OF CONTENTS

Page #

TABLE OF CONTENTS (Cont.)

Page #

INTRODUCTION

Many attempts at standardization of joint motion have been made and various methods used. The complexity of the problem precluded universal acceptance of many of these attempts.

The need for standardization was recognized by the American Academy of Orthopedic Surgeons. In 1959, a committee for the study of Joint Motion was appointed under the chairmanship of Carter R. Rowe, M.D., Boston, Mass.

The committee chose as a basis the Neutral-Zero Method described by Cave and Roberts in 1936. The modified Neutral-Zero Method was accepted in principle by the Executive Committee of the Academy in 1961. In 1962, in Vancouver, B.C., it was unanimously accepted by representatives of the Orthopedic Associations of all English-speaking countries, including Australia, Canada, Great Britian, New Zealand, South Africa and the United States. The method was also accepted by the American Society for Surgery of the Hand. In 1969, in Mexico City, it was adopted by S.I.C.O.T. (Societé Internationale de Chirurgie Orthopedique et de Traumatologie). It was adopted in Austria through the efforts of Dr. O. Russe in 1964 and was published in Switzerland by Drs. Debrunner, Mueller and Boritzy between 1968-70; and was adopted by Germany and Switzerland, where it is known as the "Null Durchgangsmethode" for reporting of disability evaluation. The Swiss Accident Insurance Company "SUVA", made it obligatory for all physicians and disability evaluators.

A different approach to standardization had been proposed by Prof. Johannes Schlaaff. He advocated universal measurements using standard application of his measuring devices, a universal recording system, and a standardization of terminology. He designed a unique fan to assure standard, one-way application of the device and to avoid errors from the source. The problem of confusion secondary to terminology and language was solved by reducing all joint motions into three basic planes designated as S: Sagittal plane, FR: Frontal plane, and ROT: Rotational plane. However, Dr. Schlaaff's use of the 360⁰ circle was impractical for clinical use. Dr. John J. Gerhardt recognized the advantages of measuring joint motion in the Neutral-Zero Method and Recording in three basic planes, thus creating the SFTR Method:(S: is Sagittal, F: is Frontal, T: is Transverse, R: is Rotation).

The SFTR Recording Method was first published in 1963 in the form of a wallchart by Dr. J. Gerhardt and the Orthopedic Equipment Company in Bourbon, Indiana, U.S.A.. Professor Otto A. Russe introduced this method in Europe and described it jointly with Dr. Gerhardt in various publications. The SFTR recording of measurement of joint motion in the Neutral-Zero Method has found a great number of followers. It was adopted as the obligatory standard method, effective January 1, 1972, by the Austrian Society of Traumatology, the Austrian Accident Insurance Company (AUVA) and all of its Traumatology Hospitals and Rehabilitation Centers, as well as the Austrian Army.

Recently, recording of strengths of agonists and antagonist muscles became possible by adding vectors to indicate direction of motion. The SFTR Recording Method provides in the shortest way possible full and precise information of joint measurements. It is simple and easily understandable by all without confusion as to discipline, language and terminology. Anyone can report measurements in the SFTR System and be immediately understood by any investigator internationally.

The data can be stored in a computer and retrieved worldwide without need for questioning or translation. SFTR documentation presents itself as an ideal recording method not only for research use, in legal medicine, Worker's Compensation, and other insurances dealing with disability claims, but also by all those dealing with dysfucntions of the musculoskeletal system, such as orthopedists, hand surgeons, rheumatologists, physiatrists, physical therapists, occupational therapists, orthotists, prosthetists, and others.

Dr. Jules Rippstein of Lausanne, Switzerland, developed the Plurimeter, which, with its simple attachments, provides the state-of-the-art precision measuring instrumentation described in the second part of this booklet.

The Plurimeter System is ideal for measuring joint motion in the SFTR Method. It allows easy, quick and more accurate measurements as compared to conventional goniometers, and secures an unsurpassed degree of reproducibility of measurements even when they are taken by different investigators.

PRINCIPLES OF MEASUREMENTS

Goniometry provides exact assessment of joint motion. The movements should be free of any active muscle contraction, which can be caused in part by reflex bracing, anxiety or fear. For this reason, the patient must be helped to relax when undergoing testing of passive or active Range of Motion. In patients who have incomplete paralytic conditions, both passive and active Range of Motion should be taken and recorded.

Changes in Range of Motion can be caused not only by surgery and injury, but may also be affected by age, sex, weather conditions, time of day, exercise, heavy workloads, etc. The above conditions should be noted in the records or reports to avoid discrepancies and wrong conclusions after follow-up evaluation by the same or different examiners.

The measurements of Range of Motion of a particular patient should be taken three times, and the average Range of Motion recorded to 5^0 increments. Reporting of increments smaller than 5^0 is neither desirable nor possible, but at times it can stop abruptly like a stop in orthotic or prosthetic devices. The documentation of the quality of motion and the kind of cessation of motion may be of significant value in prognisticating responses to therapy.

The documentation of measurements must be clear and easily readable and understandable by others in a uniform way.

THE NEUTRAL-ZERO MEASURING METHOD

The Neutral-Zero Measuring Method, known in Europe as the "Null Durch-gangsmethode", evolved as the standard measuring method because of an urgent need to facilitate communication between different investigators. The American Academy of Orthopedic Surgeons pioneered its national and international use.

Even though the Neutral-Zero Method is uniform and clear, it has the problem of lacking standard recording rules. Being language-terminology-dependent, the documented measurements cannot be read uniformly by others and there are frequent misunderstandings and misinterpretations even among investigators living in the same city and speaking the same language.

It becomes more complicated internationally: for example, the French terminology "extension gleno-humerale a partir d'un deplacement de l'humerus, retropulsion horizontal, project anterieure, abduction par rapport a la verticale et j'en passe....", is not easily understood by English- or German-speaking investigators, and the same applies to French-speaking investigators for English or German terminology.

THE SFTR-RECORDING METHOD

Introduction of the SFTR Method as an addition to the Neutral-Zero Measuring Method is a major step eliminating ambiguity of medical recording.

Dr. John J. Gerhardt of the United States developed a clear and easily understood recording system named the SFTR Method (S: is Sagittal, F: is Frontal, T: is Transverse and R: is Rotation). It is completely independent of language and terminology as it uses the universal language of numbers. Internationally, every investigator or examiner can use his or her own language and terminology when measuring, but record and communicate the findings to others in numbers. This method allows for an unsurpassed clarity, brevity and completeness of documentation. Misunderstandings and misinterpretations are completely eliminated. An additional advantage is that by virtue of its brevity and exactness it is extremely suitable for computer application.

The principles of the SFTR Method require that the motions of the joints are recorded in one of the three basic planes or parallel to them -- the Sagittal, the Frontal and Transverse planes. Using the three-numbers method of the Neutral-Zero Method, the letters "S", "F", or "T", are placed in front of the three numbers indicating the plane. The letter "R" (Rotation) is used for rototary movements as rotations can occur in any of the three planes. The three planes always relate to the body in neutral position regardless whether the actual position of the body during measurements is in standing, sitting or lying positions.

To secure uniform recording and reading, a standardized sequence of recording of the three numbers is also essential.

The number that precedes zero (0^0) always means extension, abduction or external rotation; the number following zero means flexion, adduction or internal rotation. Positions of ankyloses of joints are recorded in contrast to motions with only two numbers.

The five rules of the Standard SFTR Recording Method are described and explained in the following pages.

SFTR RECORDING

RULE 1

THE ANATOMICAL NEUTRAL-ZERO STARTING POSITION

The anatomical position of the body is the upright position with the feet facing straight forward, the arms at the side of the body and the palms facing anteriorly.

All motions begin at defined starting anatomical positions, with the exception of rotations of extremities.

The starting position for rotation is the mid-position between external and internal rotation, between supination and pronation, and between eversion and inversion.

The starting position in physiological conditions is always "zero" and is recorded as reference point in the middle as "-0-".

In pathological conditions, the motion can start in a different than physiological position and accordingly, the numbers in the middle will be different than "0". This calls immediate attention to the pathological condition.

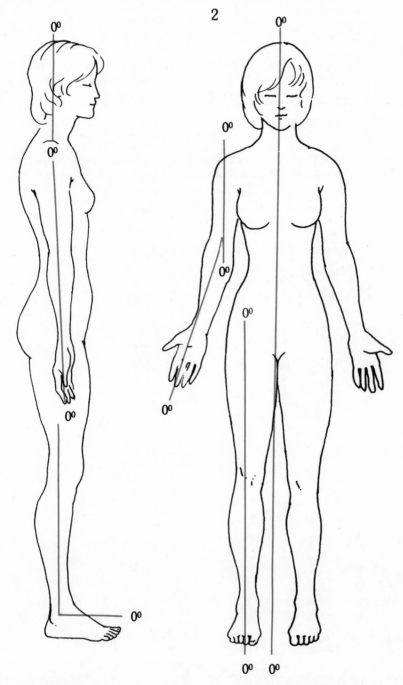

SFTR RECORDING

RULE 2

THE BASIC PLANES

To avoid confusion of terminology, all motions are recorded in three basic planes: S: is Sagittal, F: is Frontal, and T: is Transverse. All movements are reduced to motions in these three planes or planes parallel to them. They are recorded according to the plane in which the movements are performed, as S, F, and T. Rotations are recorded as R because Rotations can take place in any of the three planes.

Planes relate always to the body's anatomical position regardless of whether the subject is standing, sitting, prone or supine.

1. Measurements in the SAGITTAL plane: S
2. Measurements in the FRONTAL plane: F
3. Measurements in the TRANSVERSE plane: T
4. Measurements of ROTATION: R
5. The basic planes in the SUPINE position

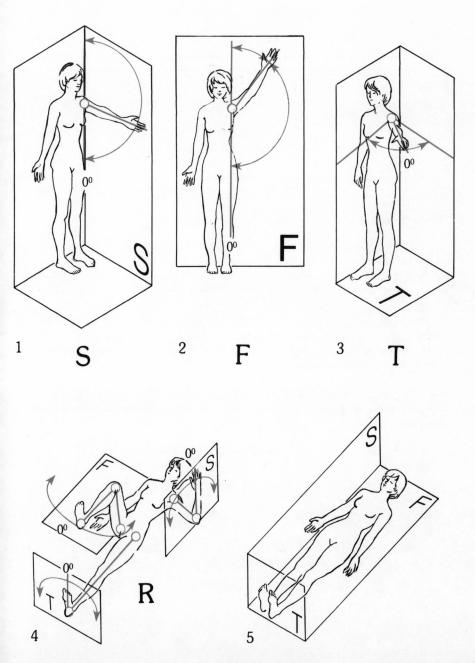

1 S

2 F

3 T

4 R

5

19

SFTR RECORDING

RULE 3

SEQUENCE OF MOTION

To secure uniform recording and reading without relying on descriptive terminology, the degrees of antagonistic motions (such as Extension and Flexion or Abduction and Adduction) have to be on the opposite sides of the Neutral-Zero.

For example:

30-0-60
(Extension-0-Flexion)

180-0-0
(Abduction-0-Adduction)

The motions are thus recorded with three numbers.

All motions are recorded with three numbers. All motions and the connotations of, *leading generally away from the middle of the body,* such as *extension, abduction, external rotation, supination, eversion* ,and motions of the head and spine to the *left,* are recorded on the *left* side of the starting position.

Motions with the connotations that are generally *leading toward the middle of the body, such as flexion, adduction, internal rotation, pronation, inversion* and motions of the head and the spine to the *right,* are recorded on the *right* side of the starting position.

This rule, combined with indication of the plane of motion by one letter, allows anyone to read and understand the recorded message in a uniform manner.

SEQUENCE OF MOTION

Plane	First (to the Left of 0) in degrees	Neutral -0- starting position	Last (to the Right of 0) in degrees
S:	Extension	-0-	Flexion
F: F: F: F: F:	Abduction Radial Deviation Elevation Valgus Side Bending of Head and Spine to the Left	-0- -0- -0- -0- -0-	Adduction Ulnar Deviation Depression Varus Side Bending of Head and Spine to the Right
T:	Horizontal Extension of Shoulder	-0-	Horizontal Flexion of Shoulder
T:	Horizontal Abduction of Hip	-0-	Horizontal Adduction of Hip
R:	External Rotation	-0-	Internal Rotation
R:	Supination of Forearm & Forefoot	-0-	Pronation of Forearm & Forefoot
R:	Eversion of Hindfoot and Midfoot	-0-	Inversion of Hindfoot and Midfoot
R:	Rotation of Head and Spine to Left	-0-	Rotation of Head and Spine to Right

SFTR RECORDING

RULE 4

LIMITATION OF MOTION

The *starting position of motion* is under normal circumstances always zero (Neutral-Zero position).

In pathological conditions, the motion can start in a different position from the anatomical Neutral-Zero starting one. Accordingly, the number recorded in the middle and representing the actual (pathological) starting position will show a number different than "0^0", calling immediate attention to the pathology.

The Neutral-Zero reference number will then be either to the left or to the right of the actual starting position, depending on the limitation of motion. In limitation of *extension*, "0" will be to the left side of the actual starting position, and in the limitation of *flexion* the "0" will be to the right.

1. Maximal extension of 60^0, motion starts at 45^0 and is recorded in the middle. There is no flexion and is recorded as 0^0

    S:60- 45-0

2. Pathological flexion deformity of the elbow of 45^0 with further flexion of 90^0 would be recorded as:

    S:0-45-90

Starting position (recorded in the middle) is not "0^0" but 45^0: there is "0" extension (recorded on the left side of the starting position), and there is further flexion to 90^0 (recorded on the right side of the starting position).

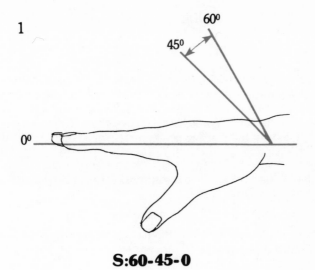

1

60⁰

45⁰

0⁰

S:60-45-0

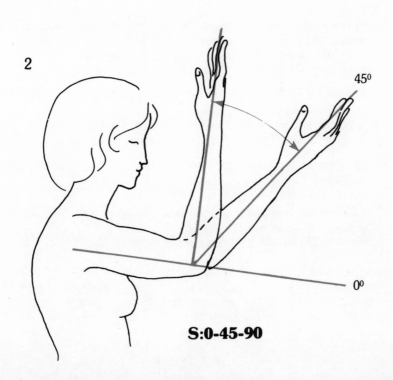

2

45⁰

0⁰

S:0-45-90

23

SFTR RECORDING

RULE 5

POSITIONS

Positions are recorded with two numbers: they are the degree of the position and the "0" starting position as reference point. The degrees of positions that are within the range of motions recorded on the left side of the starting position are placed on the left side of "0". The degrees of position within the range of motions recorded on the right side of the starting position are placed on the right side of "0".

1. The position of the wrist at 20⁰ in the extension range is recorded on the left side of Neutral-Zero. S:20-0.

2. Neutral-Zero is in the middle (as the reference point).

3. The position of the wrist at 20⁰ in the flexion range is recorded on the right of Neutral-Zero. S:0-20.

Measurements in different positions of the joint can be indicated in parentheses after recording the plane.

4. Rotation of the shoulder positioned in 90⁰ abduction (standard), can be indicated as: R(F90-0):, or for short: R(F90):
External rotation of 90⁰ and internal rotation of 90⁰,
is recorded as: R(F90):90-0-90 (red numbers in picture).

5. Rotation of shoulder with arm positioned at side of the body is recorded as: R(F0-0): or for short, R(F0):
External rotation of 45⁰ and internal rotation of 60⁰
is recorded as: R(F0):45-0-60 (red numbers in picture).

6. Rotation of shoulder with arm positioned in 60⁰ abduction and 20⁰ horizontal flexion, is recorded as:
R(F60-0, T0-20):, or for short: R(F60, T20):
External rotation of 90⁰ and internal rotation of 20⁰
in above position is recorded as:
R(F60, T20):90-0-30 (red numbers in picture).

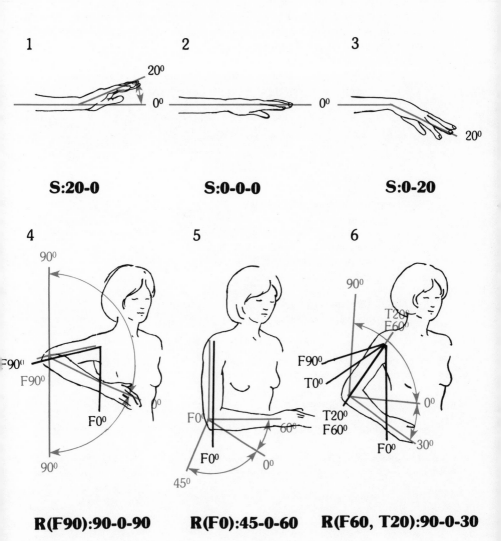

1

20°

0°

S:20-0

2

0°

S:0-0-0

3

20°

S:0-20

4

90°

F90°

F90°

F0°

0°

90°

R(F90):90-0-90

5

F0°

F0°

60°

0°

45°

R(F0):45-0-60

6

90°

T20°
F60°

F90°

T0°

T20°
F60°

F0°

0°

30°

R(F60, T20):90-0-30

SUMMARY

Knowing the five rules, we can now define all joint motion with one letter and three numbers, and any fixed joint position with one letter and two numbers. Thus, anybody familiar with the *SFTR Method* can record and read joint measurements in a uniform manner and, by means of the language of numbers, it can be understood in any language.

EXAMPLES OF *SFTR RECORDING* OF WRIST MOTIONS AND POSITIONS IN THE SAGITTAL PLANE

MEASURED MOTION	*EXTENSION-FLEXION*	*SFTR-RECORDING*
1. Neutral Position.		S:0-0-0
2. Extension of the wrist of 60⁰ and flexion of 45⁰.		S:60-0-45
3. Restricted motion of the wrist from 35⁰ of extension to 10⁰ of extension. There is no flexion.		S:35-10-0
4. Motion in the wrist is only possible from 30⁰ of extension to neutral position.		S:30-0-0
5. There is flexion *deformity* of 20⁰ and further flexion to 50⁰. There is no extension. Thus, the actual starting position is 20⁰.		S:0-20-50
6. Ankylosis of the wrist in 25⁰ of flexion.		S:0-25
7. Ankylosis of the wrist in 35⁰ of extension.		S:35-0

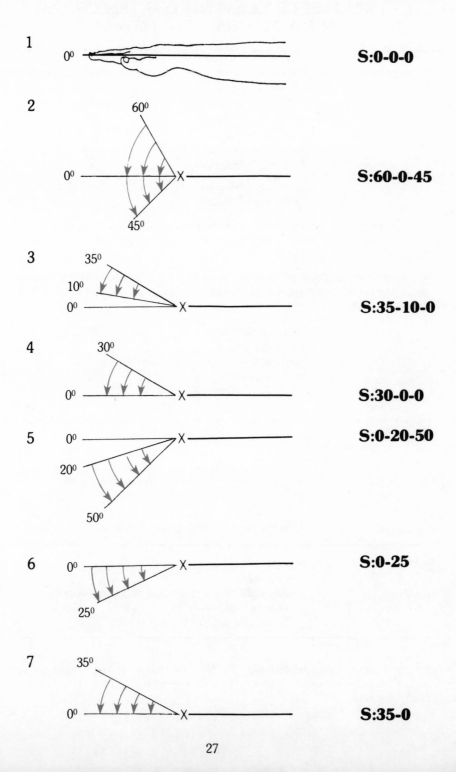

1   0⁰   **S:0-0-0**

2   60⁰
     0⁰   **S:60-0-45**
     45⁰

3   35⁰
     10⁰
     0⁰   **S:35-10-0**

4   30⁰
     0⁰   **S:30-0-0**

5   0⁰   **S:0-20-50**
     20⁰
     50⁰

6   0⁰   **S:0-25**
     25⁰

7   35⁰
     0⁰   **S:35-0**

EXAMPLES OF CONVENTIONAL RECORDING IN THE NEUTRAL-ZERO-METHOD

SHOULDER	Right	Left
Forward Flexion	70^0	170^0
Backward Extension	20^0	50^0
Abduction (active = a)	70^0	170^0
Abduction (passive = p)	80^0	170^0
Adduction (active)	30^0	75^0
Adduction (passive)	30^0	75^0
Horizontal Extension	0^0	30^0
Horizontal Flexion	0^0	100^0

Horizontal Extension on the right cannot be measured because of limited shoulder abduction. At 45^0 abduction of the right arm, the horizontal extension is 20^0 and horizontal flexion is 30^0.

External and Internal Rotation with the arm abducted at 90^0 cannot be measured on the right, and on the left the External Rotation is 60^0 and the Internal Rotation is 50^0.

	Right	Left
External Rotation with the arm at side of the body	20^0	60^0
Internal Rotation with the arm at side of the body	30^0	70^0

ELBOW
    Extension
        On the right there is limitation of extension of 30^0.
        On the left there is hyperextension of 5^0.
    Flexion
        On the right, flexion starts at 30^0 and there is further flexion to 90^0, and on the left the flexion is 150^0.

FOREARM
    Supination
        The right forearm is fixed in 20^0 supination.
        The supination on the left is 90^0.
        The pronation on the left is 80^0.

In conventional recording, lengthy description is necessary to define pathological conditions (ankylosis, limitation of motion, etc). It is not suitable for computer use.

EXAMPLES OF SFTR RECORDING OF SAME MEASUREMENTS

SHOULDER		Right	Left
	S:	20-0-70	50-0-170
	Fa:	70-0-30	170-0-75
	Fp:	80-0-30	170-0-75
	T:	0	30-0-100
	T(F45):	20-0-30	
	R(F90):	0	60-0-50
	R(F0):	20-0-30	60-0-70

ELBOW	S:0-30-90	5-0-150

FOREARM	R:20-0	90-0-80

In the SFTR-Recording, all information is documented in a simple, precise and consise form without lengthy description or confusion as to discipline, language, and terminology. It is ideal for computer storage and analysis.

ENGLISH TERMINOLOGY OF COMMONLY MEASURED JOINTS

JOINTS

Joints of the spine and head
  temporo-mandibular
  atlanto-occipital
  cervical spine
  thoracic spine
  lumbar spine
  lumbo-sacral joint

Shoulder girdle joints
  acromio-clavicular joint
  sterno-clavicular joint

Upper extremity joints
  shoulder joint
  gleno-humeral joint
  elbow joint
  humero-ulnar joint
  humero-radial joint
  proximal and distal radio-ulnar joints

Hand joints
  radio-carpal joint
  carpal joints
  ulno-menisco-triquetral joint
  carpo-metacarpal joints
  carpo-metacarpal joint óf the thumb
  intermetacarpal joints
  metacarpo-phalangeal joints
  interphalangeal joints of the hand

Pelvic girdle joints
  sacroiliac joint
  pubic symphysis

Lower extremity joints
  hip joint
  knee joint
  tibio-fibular joint
  tibio-fibular syndesmosis
  talo-crural joint (upper ankle joint)

Foot joints

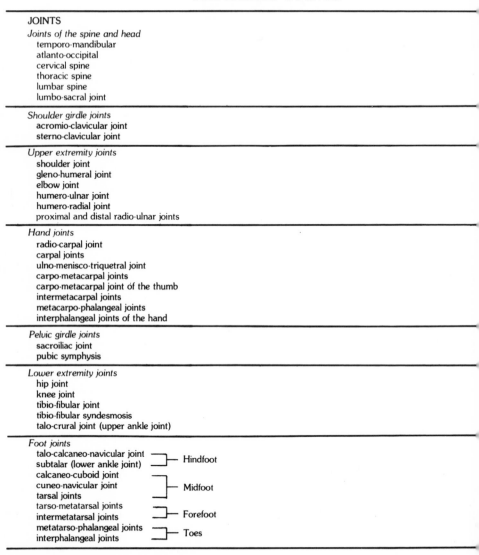

  talo-calcaneo-navicular joint ⎤
  subtalar (lower ankle joint)   ⎦— Hindfoot
  calcaneo-cuboid joint ⎤
  cuneo-navicular joint ├— Midfoot
  tarsal joints ⎦
  tarso-metatarsal joints ⎤
  intermetatarsal joints ⎦— Forefoot
  metatarso-phalangeal joints ⎤
  interphalangeal joints ⎦— Toes

Right (Rt)   Left (Lt)

For international use, the measured joint should be indicated in Latin according to the standardized **NOMINA ANATOMICA** terminology.

INTERNATIONAL-LATIN-TERMINOLOGY OF SAME JOINTS

ARTICULATIONES

Articulationes columnae vertebralis et cranii
   articulatio temporomandibularis
   articulatio atlanto-occipitalis
   articulationes columnae vertebralis cervicalis
   articulationes columnae vertebralis thoracalis
   articulationes columnae vertebralis lumbalis
   articulatio lumbosacralis

Articulationes cinguli membri superioris
   articulatio acromio-clavicularis
   articulatio sterno-clavicularis

Articulationes membris superioris liberi
   articulatio humeri
   articulatio gleno-humeri
   articulatio cubiti
   articulatio humero-ulnaris
   articulatio humero radialis
   articulatio radio-ulnaris proximalis et distalis

Articulationes manus
   articulatio radio-carpea
   articulationes intercarpeae
   articulatio ulno-menisco-triquetris
   articulationes carpo-metacarpeae
   articulatio carpometacarpea pollicis
   articulationes intermetacarpeae
   articulationes metacarpo-phalangeae
   articulationes interphalangeae manus

Articulationes cinguli membri inferioris
   articulatio sacro-iliaca
   symphysis pubica

Articulationes membri inferioris liberi
   articulatio coxae
   articulatio genus
   articulatio tibio-fibularis
   syndesmosis tibio-fibularis
   articulatio talo-cruralis

Articulationes pedis
   articulatio talo-calcaneo-navicularis
   articulatio subtalaris ⎤— Pars posterior pedis
   articulatio calcaneo-cuboidea ⎤
   articulatio cuneo-navicularis ⎥— Pars media pedis
   articulationes intertarseae
   articulationes tarso-metatarseae ⎤— Pars anterior pedis
   articulationes intermetatarseae ⎦
   articulationes metatarso-phalangeae ⎤
   articulationes interphalangeae pedis ⎦— Digiti (phalanges)

Dexter (Dext.)   Sinister (Sin.)

From: Nomina Anatomica, Fourth Edition, Excerpta Medica,
          Amsterdam, Oxford, 1977

THE INTERNATIONAL STANDARD
SFTR POCKET GONIOMETER

The Standard Pocket Goniometer is a handy device to facilitate measurements in the Neutral-Zero-Method and standard SFTR recordings. The *values* are *generally* indicated by the *black arrow*. Motions of the *shoulder* are read at the *black triangle*, and those of the *ankle joint* at the *red arrow*.

THE INTERNATIONAL STANDARD SFTR GONIOMETER

The International Standard SFTR Goniometer is also a two-armed goniometer for clinic or hospital use: its large dimensions enable the examiner to take more accurate measurements and readings. It contains three scales: 0^0 to 180^0, 0^0 to 90^0, and 180^0 to 360^0, as well as inches and centimeter scales.

APPLICATION OF THE GONIOMETERS

The arms of the Goniometer are placed over or parallel to the long mechanical axes of the structures that define the angle of the joint. True axes of rotation of joints often vary in different positions of the joint and are difficult to determine. Therefore, placement of the rotational axis of the Goniometer can only be approximate, and the examiner must concentrate on accurate application of the arms. For details, refer to tables later in this book. (18,19)

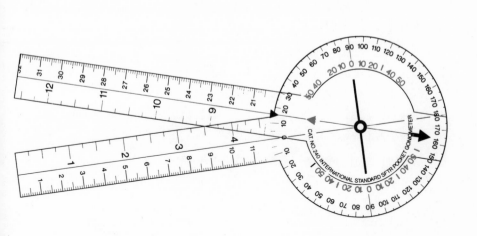

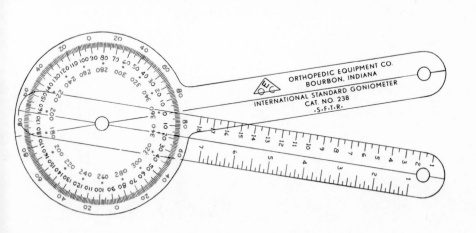

EXAMPLES OF APPLICATION OF THE GONIOMETER

S-MOTION

1. Extension and flexion of shoulder.
2. Flexion of elbow.
3. Extension (dorsiflexion) and flexion of wrist.
4. Flexion of hip.
5. Flexion of knee.
6. Extension (dorsiflexion) and flexion of ankle.

R-MOTION

7. *Rotation of head* (cervical spine):
   The fixed arm of the goniometer is placed in the frontal plane, the movable arm follows the rotation of the head using the occipito-nasal line (sagittal suture) as indicator of motion. Read on red 0-90 scale.

8. *Rotation of shoulder in 90⁰ abduction:*
   The fixed arm of the goniometer is placed parallel to the lateral axillary line, the movable arm parallel to the lateral midline of the ulna which serves as indicator of motion. Read on red 0-90 scale.

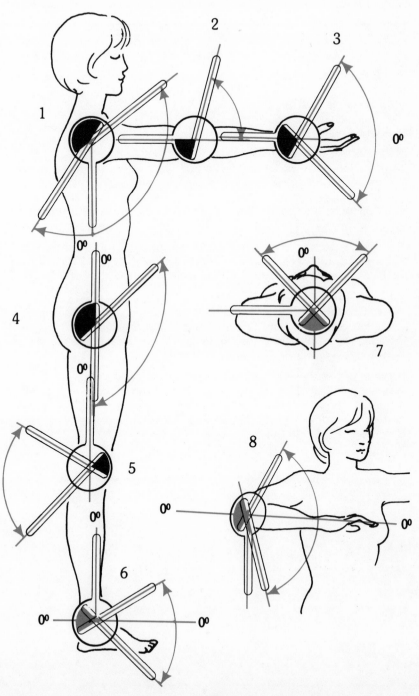

1

2

3

0⁰

4

0⁰

0⁰

0⁰

5

0⁰

6

0⁰

0⁰

7

0⁰

8

0⁰

0⁰

35

MEASUREMENTS OF THE SHOULDER GIRDLE
AND SHOULDER

SHOULDER GIRDLE

1. Elevation (upward motion) and depression (downward motion) of the shoulder, may also be measured in degrees in "F" however, these motions are rarely measured with the conventional goniometer (see page 74/75).

2. Retraction and protraction of the shoulder girdle are primary motions of the scapula and the clavicle. They are measured in "T" from the "0" starting position as illustrated.

SHOULDER

3. *Motion of the shoulder in S.*
   Shoulder extension of 45^0 and flexion of 170^0 (also called posterior and anterior elevation) is performed in the sagittal plane and simply recorded as: S:45-0-170.
   Read values at the black triangle when using the Pocket Goniometer.

4. *Motion of the shoulder in F.*
   Shoulder abduction of 180^0 and adduction of 45^0 (in front of the body) is performed in the frontal plane and recorded as F:180-0-45. Read values at the black triangle when using the Pocket Goniometer.

5. *Motion of the shoulder in T.*
   Horizontal extension of 45^0 and horizontal flexion (also called horizontal abduction and adduction) is performed in the transverse plane at 90^0 of shoulder abduction and recorded as T:45-0-135. Read values at the black triangle when using the Pocket Goniometer.

6. *Rotation of the shoulder with arm in 90^0 Abduction.*
   External rotation of the shoulder of 90^0 and internal rotation of 90^0 with arm in 90^0 abduction, elbow in 90^0 flexion and forearm used as indicator of motion, is recorded as R(F90):90-0-90. Read values at the black triangles when using the Pocket Goniometer.

ARTICULATIONES CINGULI MEMBRI SUPERIORIS
ARTICULATIO HUMERI

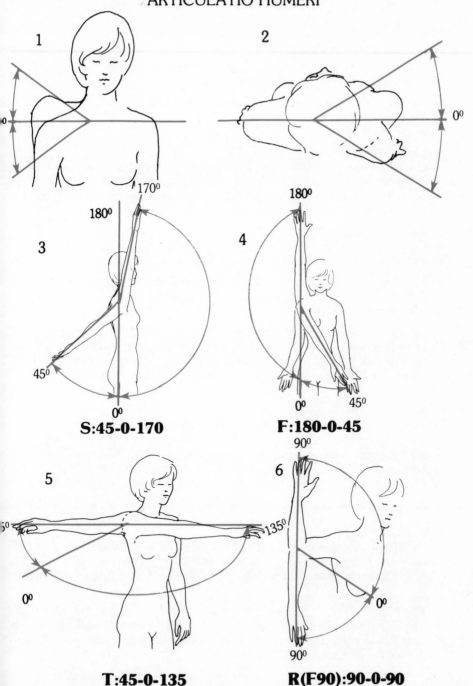

1

2

0^0

0^0

170^0

180^0

3

45^0

0^0

S:45-0-170

180^0

4

0^0

45^0

F:180-0-45

90^0

5

0^0

135^0

T:45-0-135

6

0^0

90^0

90^0

R(F90):90-0-90

MEASUREMENTS OF THE ELBOW AND WRIST

THE ELBOW

1. *Extension and Flexion*
   The normal range of motion of the elbow with only flexion from the Zero Starting Position is noted as S:0-0-145

2. *Hyperextension is an excessive motion* beyond the Zero Starting Position. If hyperextension is 10^0, the total range is recorded as S:10-0-145. Read values at the black arrow.

3. *Limitation of Motion.*
   Limitation of elbow motion with lack of extension of 30^0, further flexion to 90^0 and lack of flexion beyond 90^0, the total range of motion being only 60^0, is recorded as S:0-30-90. (There is no hyperextension, the actual starting point is not zero but 30^0 of flexion and further flexion is possible to 90^0.)

   Positional Deformities
   Cubitus Valgus and Cubitus Varus.
   The elbow has a physiological valgus position averaging 10^0. F:10-0

4. *Unstable elbow* (flail joint). There is abnormal mobility in the frontal plane, and valgus position of 10^0 may be increased passively to 20^0.
   Recording: F:20-10-0.

5. *Right elbow with varus deformity of 10^0 (cubitus varus).* There is not only lack of normal valgus of 10^0, but additional 10^0 of varus producing total pathological angulation; namely, varus of 20^0. Recording of pathological position is: F:0-20. (Average normal elbow position would be: F:10-0).

6. *Rotation of the Forearm.*
   Starting Zero Position (neutral rotation) is present when the dorsum of the hand is parallel to the long axis of the arm with the elbow flexed 90^0 and close to the body. Supination of the forearm of 90^0 and pronation of 90^0 is recorded as R:90-0-90. If supination is limited to 45^0, and pronation to 50^0, the recording is R:45-0-50. Read values as usual at the black arrow.

THE WRIST

7. *Extension and Flexion.*
   Extension (dorsiflexion) of 50^0 and flexion of 60^0 is recorded S:50-0-60, "0" being the neutral position of the wrist with the hand parallel to the long axis of the forearm. Read values at the black arrow of the Pocket Goniometer.

8. *Radial and Ulnar Deviation.*
   The Neutral-Zero Position is present when the fc.   .n and the third metacarpal are in line. Radial deviation of 20^0 (abduction with the palm of the hand facing anteriorly in the anatomical position), and ulnar deviation of 30^0 (adduction) is recorded as F:20-0-30.

ARTICULATIO CUBITI, RADIO-CARPEA ET RADIO-ULNARIS DISTALIS

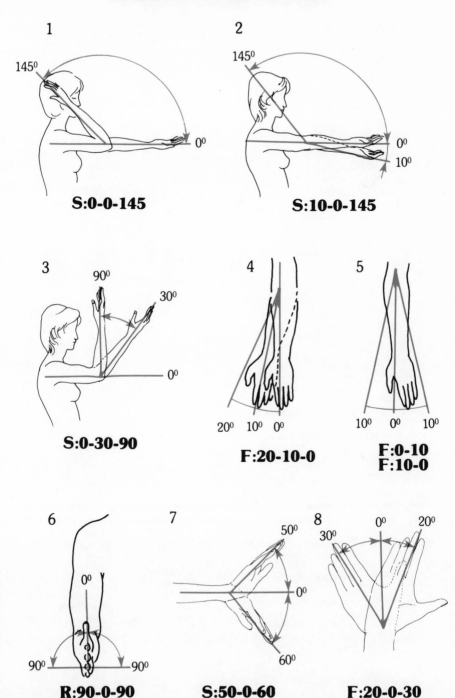

1
145°
0°
S:0-0-145

2
145°
0°
10°
S:10-0-145

3
90°
30°
0°
S:0-30-90

4
20° 10° 0°
F:20-10-0

5
10° 0° 10°
F:0-10
F:10-0

6
0°
90° 90°
R:90-0-90

7
50°
0°
60°
S:50-0-60

8
0° 20°
30°
F:20-0-30

39

TERMINOLGY OF THE HAND

1. Rascetta, prox. skin fold
2. Ulna
3. Styloid process of ulna
4. Lunate
5. Triquetrum
6. Pisiform
7. Hamate
8. Capitate
9. Metacarpal V
   (Head, MC V)
10. Proximal phalanx V
    (Base, PP V)
11. Proximal phalanx V
    (Shaft, PP V)
12. Proximal phalanx V
    (Head, PP V)
13. Proximal interphalangeal joint V
    (PIP V)
14. Middle phalanx V (PM V)
15. Distal interphalang. joint V
    (DIP V)
16. Distal phalanx V (PD V)

17. Head of middle phalanx IV
    (Head, PM IV)
18. Distal phalanx III (PD III)
19. Distal phalanx II (PD II)
20. Distal interphalang. joint II
    (DIP II)
21. Prox. interphalangeal joint II
    (PIP II)
22. Metacarpo-phalangeal joint II
    (MCP II)
23. Distal phalanx I (PD I)
24. Interphalangeal joint I (IPP)
25. Proximal phalanx I (PP I)
26. Sesamoid
27. Metacarpo-phalang. joint I (MCP I)
28. Metacarpals I-V
29. Trapezoid
30. Trapezium
31. Scaphoid
32. Styloid process of radius
33. Restricta, distal skin fold
34. Radius

A. Terminology of the hand: shaded areas on skeletal parts are visible or palpable under the skin.

B. First ray of the hand.
   DP I   distal phalanx
   PP I   proximal phalanx
   MC I   metacarpal
   IPP   interphalangeal joint of the thumb
   MCP I   metacarpophalangeal joint
   CMC I   carpometacarpal joint

C. Second to fifth ray of the hand.
   DP   distal phalanx
   MP   middle phalanx
   PP   proximal phalanx
   MC   metacarpal
   DIP   distal interphalangeal joint
   PIP   proximal interphalang. joint
   MCP   metacarpophalangeal joint
   CMC   carpometacarpal joint

D. a-a Axis of hand (through third metacarpal and middle finger).

   I   thumb (first digit)
   II   index finger (second digit)
   III middle finger (third digit)
   IV   ring finger (fourth digit)
   V   little finger (fifth digit)
   1   carpal joints
   2   radiocarpal joints
   3   distal radio-ulnar joint and ulno-menisco-triquetral j◖

E.

1. Distal interphal. skin crease.
2. Prox. interphal. skin crease.
3. Palmar digital skin crease.
4. Distal palmar crease.
5. Proximal palmar crease.
6. Ulnar crease.
7. Median crease.
8. Wrist crease (prox.-rascetta, dist.-restricta).
9. Distal skin crease of the thumb.
10. Thenar crease.

TERMINOLOGIA MANUS

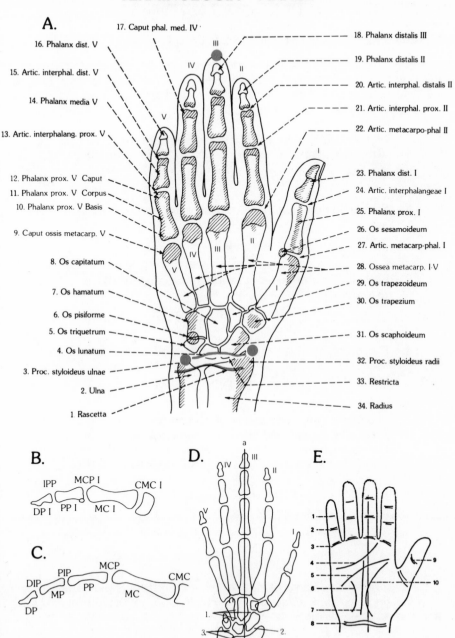

A.

17. Caput phal. med. IV

16. Phalanx dist. V

15. Artic. interphal. dist. V

14. Phalanx media V

13. Artic. interphalang. prox. V

12. Phalanx prox. V Caput
11. Phalanx prox. V Corpus
10. Phalanx prox. V Basis

9. Caput ossis metacarp. V

8. Os capitatum

7. Os hamatum

6. Os pisiforme

5. Os triquetrum

4. Os lunatum

3. Proc. styloideus ulnae

2. Ulna

1. Rascetta

18. Phalanx distalis III

19. Phalanx distalis II

20. Artic. interphal. distalis II

21. Artic. interphal. prox. II

22. Artic. metacarpo-phal II

23. Phalanx dist. I
24. Artic. interphalangeae I

25. Phalanx prox. I

26. Os sesamoideum

27. Artic. metacarp-phal. I

28. Ossea metacarp. I·V

29. Os trapezoideum

30. Os trapezium

31. Os scaphoideum

32. Proc. styloideus radii

33. Restricta

34. Radius

B.

IPP MCP I CMC I
DP I PP I MC I

C.

DIP PIP MCP CMC
DP MP PP MC

D.

E.

41

MEASUREMENTS OF THE HAND
DIGITS 2-5 (Long Fingers)

MEASUREMENTS OF THE DIGITS 2-5 (Long Fingers)

The Neutral-Zero Starting Position when recording motions or positions of the long fingers is the position of full extension of the fingers which are aligned with the metacarpals. Hyperextension is recorded to the left of -0- and the value of maximal possible flexion to the right.

1. Motion in the metacarpophalangeal joints of the fingers with no hyperextension and flexion to 90^0 is recorded as:

   MCP   S:0-0-90

2. Same motion but with 30^0 of hyperextension is recorded as:

   MCP   S:30-0-90

3. Flexion in the proximal interphalangeal joints of 100^0 is recorded as:

   PIP   S:0-0-100

4. Flexion of 45^0 in the distal interphalangeal joints is recorded as:

   DIP   S:0-0-45

5. Functional measurements of abduction-adduction. Fingers are maximally spread, and distances measured between finger-tips as illustrated. Hand span: the distance from the tip of thumb to the tip of the little finger of a spread hand (I-V).

6. Hyperextension of distal interphalangeal joint of 15^0 with flexion to 45^0 is recorded as:

   DIP   S:15-0-45

Remarks:
Measurements of Range of Motion of thumb and fingers should be done with a special finger goniometer such as the PLURI-DIG, to assure proper application and accurate readings.

MANUS
ARTICULATIONES DIGITI I-V

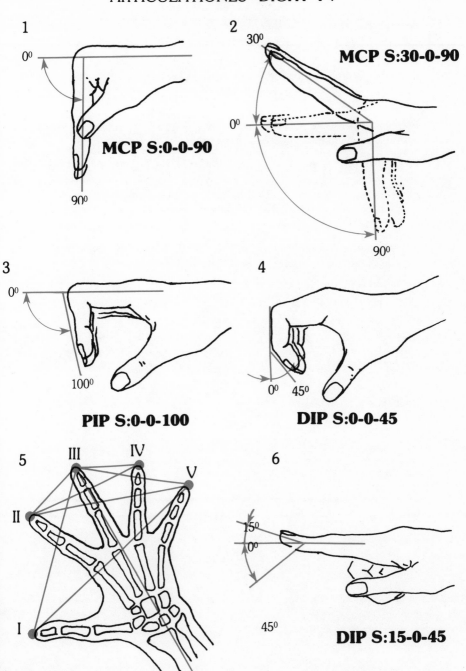

1
0⁰
90⁰
MCP S:0-0-90

2
30⁰
MCP S:30-0-90
0⁰
90⁰

3
0⁰
100⁰
PIP S:0-0-100

4
0⁰ 45⁰
DIP S:0-0-45

5
III IV V II I

6
15⁰
0⁰
45⁰
DIP S:15-0-45

43

MEASUREMENTS OF THE HAND

FUNCTIONAL MEASUREMENTS OF THE FINGERS
MEASUREMENTS OF THE CARPO-METACARPAL JOINT I (CMC I)

1. Impaired overall extension of a finger can be measured functionally by recording the distance between the tip of the finger and the plane of the dorsum of the hand.

2. Impaired overall flexion of a finger is measured by recording the fingertip to palm distance (fingernail to palm).

3. The two axes of the carpo-metacarpal joint I (saddle joint), are at 90^0 angle to each other and about 45^0 to the plane of the palm. To simplify measurements, the motions are divided into two components or vectors and measured in the sagittal (S) and frontal (F) planes. The motions are recorded as VS and VF respectively.

4. Palmar abduction-adduction in the CMC I joint is measured in the sagittal plane and is recorded as: CMC I VS:60-0-0

5. Radial abduction-adduction in the CMC I joint is measured in the frontal plane and recorded as: CMC I VF:40-0-15.

MANUS
ARTICULATIO CARPO-METACARPEAE I

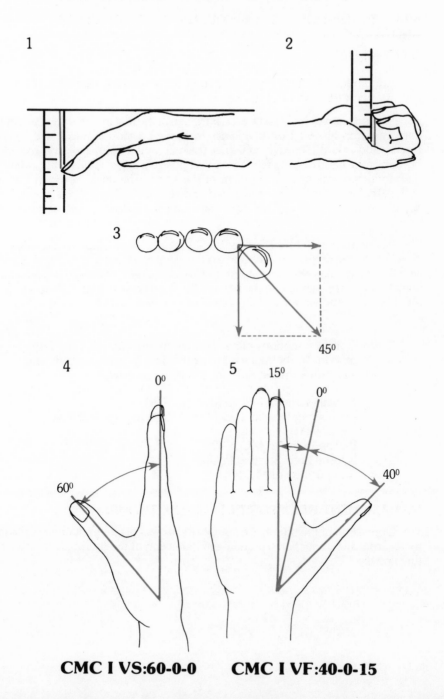

CMC I VS:60-0-0   **CMC I VF:40-0-15**

MEASUREMENTS OF THE THUMB

MEASUREMENT OF CARPOMETACARPAL JOINT I (CMC I) AND THUMB

CIRCUMDUCTION

Circumduction of the first metacarpal is the complete motion of MC I from Retroposition through Neutral-Zero to Anteposition.

Anteposition of MC I is the arcuar motion of the first metacarpal solely at the carpometacarpal joint I (saddle joint), from the position of maximal extension (radial abduction), through maximal (palmar abduction), towards the ulnar border of the hand, maintaining the widest possible angle between the extended and abducted thumb and the palm of the hand. The angle between the first metacarpal and the palm is measured and recorded. The palm is stabilized in supination on the table with MC I and the thumb extended beyond the edge of the table.

Retroposition of MC I is the continuation of opposition in the opposite direction, as the first metacarpal passes the plane of the palm of the hand dorsally with the thumb maximally extended (radially abducted). The angle between MC I in maximal retroposition and the palm of the hand is measured. Retroposition of MC I is measured with the palm stabilized in prone position on the table.

1. Complex motions of the first metacarpal and thumb. True motions in the metacarpal joint I (saddle joint) are indicated with black, measured motions with red arrows.

2. Measurements of circumduction (CR):
   the average normal R.O.M. is 20-0-90 and recorded as:
   CR:20-0-90.
   Retroposition of MC I: 20^0
   Neutral-Zero Starting Position,
   Anteposition of MC I: 90^0

MEASUREMENT OF OPPOSITION OF THE THUMB

Opposition of the thumb is a composite motion of circumduction of the first metacarpal and abduction, rotation and extension of the thumb. It is measured functionally.

POLLEX
ARTICULATIO CARPO-METACARPEAE I

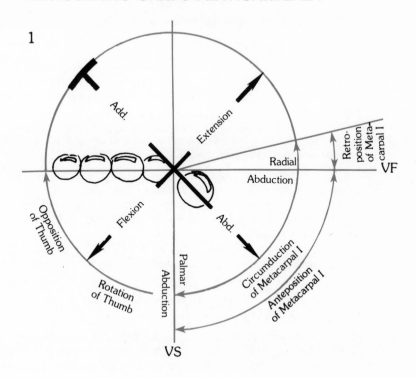

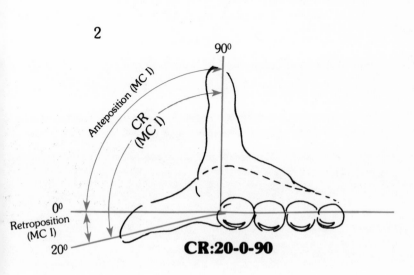

CR:20-0-90

MEASUREMENTS OF THE THUMB

MEASUREMENTS OF OPPOSITION AND ROTATION OF THE THUMB

1-3 Opposition of the thumb is achieved by a combination of circumduction of the first metacarpal and abduction, rotation and extension of the thumb. Circumduction, Extension and Abduction are described on preceding pages.

2-4 The drawing represents functional measurements of the opposition of the first metacarpal. (see pages 46/47).

MC I opposition is recorded by measuring the distance in cm between the midpoint of the distal crease of the thumb and the point of intersection of the long axis of the third metacarpal and the distal palmar crease, with the first metacarpal in maximal circumduction and full extension of the joints of the thumb.

Opposition of the thumb is measured functionally (see page 50/51).

3. Rotation of the thumb may be recorded by measuring the difference between the angles the thumbnail makes with the plane of the palm at beginning and end of opposition.

Pinch movements as performed between the thumb and fingers are composite motions and include circumduction of the thumb ray, and appropriate flexion or extension of the metacarpo-phalangeal interphalangeal joints. This must be distinguished from true opposition. Functional measurements of pinch movements are presented on page 50/51.

5. Measuring of extension component of thumb opposition.

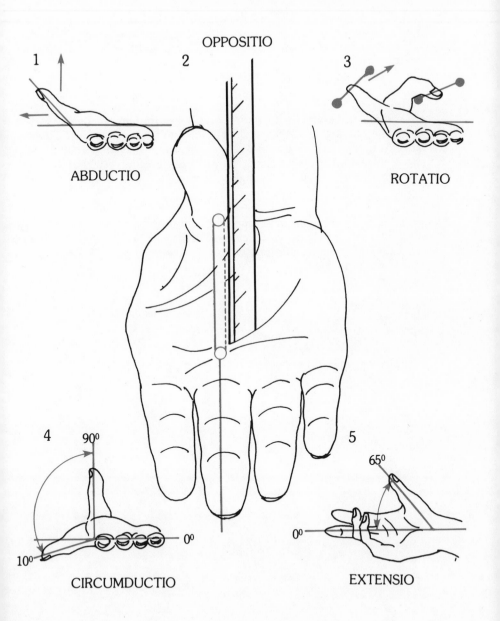

OPPOSITIO

1 ABDUCTIO

3 ROTATIO

4 CIRCUMDUCTIO

5 EXTENSIO

MEASUREMENTS OF THE THUMB

1. Neutral-Zero Starting Position when measuring motions of the thumb is the fully extended thumb. Flexion in the metacarpophalangeal joint (MCP I) of 60^0 and the interphalangeal joint of the thumb (IPP)of 65^0 with no hyper-extension is noted as:

    MCP I S:0-0-60   IPP S:0-0-65

2. *Functional measurement* of thumb and finger motion are generally easier and more practical. Impairment of thumb motion is expressed by the distance from the tip of the thumb to the metacarpophalangeal joint of the little finger, measured in centimeters. The ruler is placed vertically to the palm. The arm of the goniometer contains a centimeter gradation.

3,4. *Functional measurements* of impaired motion of the thumb is often rerorded by measuring the distance from the tip of the thumb to the tip of the distal, the proximal interphalangeal joints and the metacarpophalangeal joint of the little finger.

Abbreviations:
MCP   Metacarpophalangeal joint
PIP   Proximal interphalangeal joint
IPP   Interphalangeal joint of the pollex
AD   Apex digiti (tip of finger at fingernail)

POLLEX
ARTICULATIO METACARPOPHALANGEAE I ET INTERPHALANGEAE POLLICIS
MENSURAE FUNCTIONALES

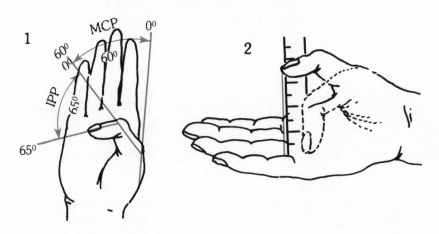

MCP I S:0-0-60

IPP   S:0-0-65

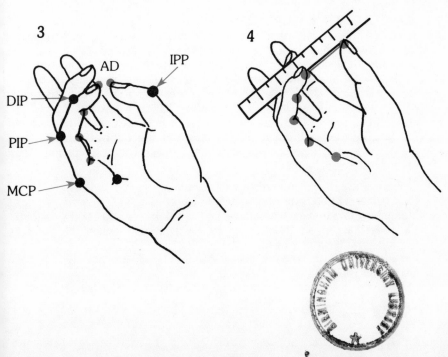

MEASUREMENTS OF THE SPINE

MEASUREMENTS OF THE CERVICAL SPINE

Conventional measurements of the cervical spine cannot be taken accurately because of paucity of landmarks. They are not readily reproducible. (Refer to Plurimeter measurements on page 80,81,82 and 83).

1. Attempt of measurements of extension-flexion using a conventional goniometer.

2. Using a tongue blade held between teeth at an angle to increase accuracy of measurements of flexion and extension.

MEASUREMENTS OF THE THORACIC AND LUMBAR SPINE

3.4 For accurate measurements of kyphosis or lordosis, only special instruments such as the Kyphometer of Debrunner or the Plurimeter (see page 82-83) can be used. Clinical measurements of scoliosis are never correct and should be measured only on X-rays using the Cobbs Method (see pages 70-71).

5. Rotation of the thoracic spine with the patient in sitting position. Rotation to the left is recorded first and rotation to the right last. Average.R.O.M. is: R:45-0-45

6. Alternative method of extension of the thoracic spine and lumbar spine with patient in prone position.

7,8. FUNCTIONAL MEASUREMENTS
A flexible plastic or metal tape is applied as illustrated, and the distance between spinal processes of C7 and S1 are measured with the patient in an upright position. Another reading is taken in maximal flexion (forward bending) of the spine. As the patient flexes the spine, the measured distance will increase because the spinal processes spread apart. An average increase of 10 cm is found in the adult, 2.5 cm between C7 and T12 and 7 cm between T12 and S1. Another useful and widely accepted method for functional measurement of the spine is the detirmination of the fingertip-leg and fingertip-floor distance. Knees of the patient must be extended during the test.

9,10. Occiput -- wall distance (limited extension).
Chin -- sternal notch distance (limited flexion).
Maximum lumbar spine -- wall distance (variations of lordosis). (Distal fold)
Earlobe -- acromion distance in maximal lateral bending of cervical spine (lateral tilt of the head).
Fingertip -- floor distance in maximal lateral bending of the spine to the left and to the right.

COLUMNA VERTEBRALIS

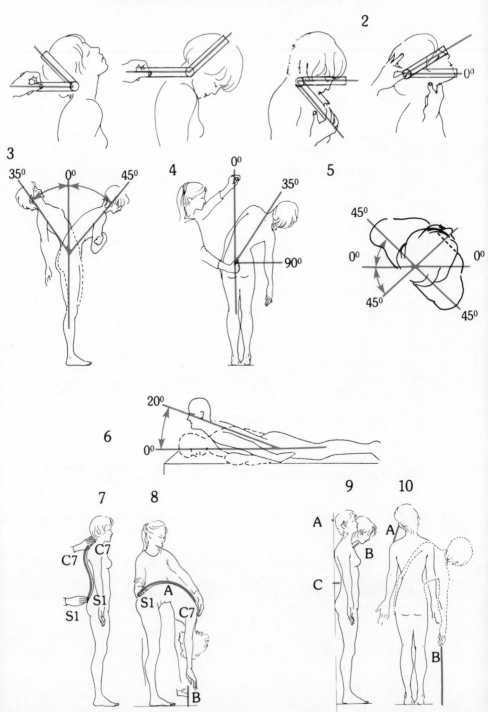

MEASUREMENTS OF THE HIP

MEASUREMENTS OF THE HIP

EXTENSION-FLEXION

1. Extension is measured in the prone position with the opposite hip flexed over the edge of the table. It is used only for evaluation of passive motion of hip and lumbar spine combined.

2. Flexion is measured in the supine position. The opposite hip is extended. Pelvis and spine must be immobilized. The Thomas maneuver is used to detect hip flexion contracture.

Combined motion presented in Figures 1 and 2 is recorded as: S:15-0-120.

ROTATION

Measurements are taken in a standing or preferably sitting or supine position. The leg is the indicator of motion: it moves medially with external rotation and laterally with internal rotation of the hip. External rotation is always recorded first and internal rotation last.

3. External Rotation of the hip of 45^0 and internal rotation of 45^0 with the hip and knee flexed 90^0 is recorded as: R(S90, S90):45-0-45.

4. External rotation of the hip of 45^0 and internal rotation of 40^0 with the hip and knee extended is recorded as: R(S0, S0):45-0-40.

Measurements are taken in supine position. Abduction is noted first and adduction last. In testing adduction of one extremity, the other must be lifted out of the way and supported passively.

ABDUCTION AND ADDUCTION

5. There is an abduction deformity on the right: the motion starts at 10^0 of abduction and further abduction is possible to 45^0; there is no adduction and the starting position is 10^0 (noted in the middle). SFTR recording is F:45-10-0.

ADDUCTION CONTRACTURE

6. There is no abduction. Motion is from 0^0 to 35^0 adduction. SFTR-Recording is F:0-0-35.

When measuring abduction and adduction of the hip, the pelvis must be stabilized. The stationary arm of the goniometer is placed over the line connecting the left and right iliac spines. The movable arm is on or parallel to the long axis of the measured thigh.

ARTICULATIO COXAE

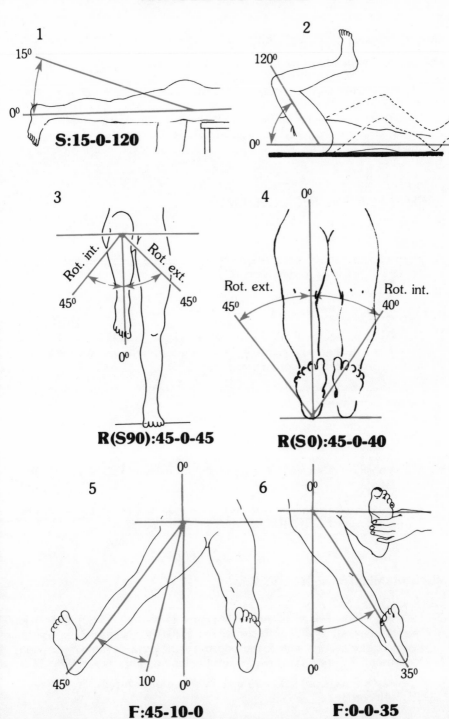

1
15⁰
0⁰
S:15-0-120

2
120⁰
0⁰

3
Rot. int.   Rot. ext.
45⁰   45⁰
0⁰
R(S90):45-0-45

4
0⁰
Rot. ext.   Rot. int.
45⁰   40⁰
R(S0):45-0-40

5
0⁰
45⁰   10⁰   0⁰
F:45-10-0

6
0⁰
0⁰   35⁰
F:0-0-35

MEASUREMENTS OF THE KNEE, ANKLE

MEASUREMENTS OF THE KNEE
HYPEREXTENSION-FLEXION

1. Normally there is no hyperextension and knee flexion of 130^0 is recorded as: S:0-0-130.
    Hyperextension of 10^0 and flexion of 130^0 is recorded as: S:10-0-130. The arms of the goniometer are applied laterally to the long axes of the thigh and the leg.

FLEXED KNEE (GENU ANTECURVATUM)
BACK KNEE (GENU RECURVATUM)

2. Figure 2 shows flexion contracture with inability to extend the knee of 10^0. SFTR-Recording is: S:0-10.

3. Figure 3 shows back knee deformity with hyperextension of the knee joint of 10^0.   SFTR-Recording is: S:10-0.

KNOCK KNEES, (GENUA VALGA)

4. Normal or pathological angulation between femur and tibia may be determined exactly by X-ray. Figure 4 shows valgus position with supplementary angle of 25^0. SFTR recording is: F:25-0.

    Functional measurements: with knees close together distance of medial malleoli is measured in cm.

BOW LEGS (GENUA VARA)

5. Varus position of knees with supplementary angle of 25^0. SFTR recording is: F:0-25.

    Functional measurements: with feet close together, the distance between the medial aspect of the left and right knee is measured in cm.

MEASUREMENTS OF THE ANKLE
EXTENSION-FLEXION

6. Extension (dorsiflexion of the ankle joint -- talocrural), of 20^0 and flexion (plantar flexion) of 50^0 is recorded as S:20-0-50. Neutral-Zero Starting Position: foot at right angle to the long axis of the leg (as in standing position). Measurements are usually taken with the hip and knee flexed 90^0.

7. Heel varus (inversion) left and right. (Valgus not pictured). SFTR-Recording: F:0-10.

ARTICULATIO GENUS ET TALO-CALCANEI

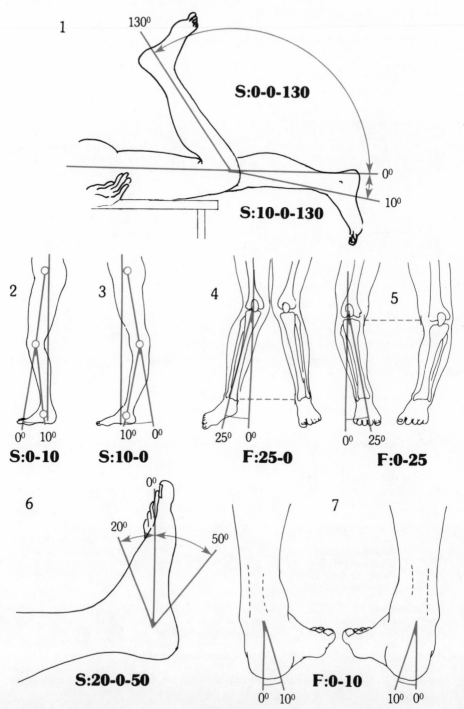

1   130⁰

S:0-0-130

0⁰

10⁰

S:10-0-130

2   0⁰   10⁰   **S:0-10**

3   10⁰   0⁰   **S:10-0**

4   25⁰   0⁰   **F:25-0**

5   0⁰   25⁰   **F:0-25**

6   0⁰   20⁰   50⁰   **S:20-0-50**

7   **F:0-10**   0⁰ 10⁰   10⁰ 0⁰

TERMINOLOGY OF THE FOOT

A. 1. Distal interphalangeal joint IV
       (DIP IV)
   2. Prox. interphalang. joint IV
       (PIP IV)
   3. Distal phalanx V (PD V)
   4. Middle phalanx V (PM V)
   5. Prox. phalanx V (PP V)
   6. Metatarso-phal. joint V (MTP V)
   7. Metatarsal V
       (Head, MT V)
   8. Metatarsal V
       (Shaft, MT V)
   9. Tuberosity of metatarsal V
       (MT V)
   10. Metatarsal V
       (Basis, MT V)
   11. Tarso-metatarsal joint V (TMT V)
   12. Cuboid
   13. Calcaneus
   14. Lat. malleolus
   15. Fibula

HINDFOOT (PPP)
   16. Tibia
   17. Med.malleolus
   18. Talus
   19. Chopart line

MIDFOOT (PMP)
   20. Navicular
   21. Cuneiforms
       medial
       intermediate
       lateral
   22. Lisfranc line

FOREFOOT (PAP)
   23. 1st metatarsal (MT I) Base
   24. 1st metatarsal (MT I) Shaft
   25. 1st metatarsal (MT I) Head
   26. Metatarso-phalangeal line

TOES
   27. Metatarso-phalangeal joint I
       (MTP I)
   28. Prox. phalanx I (PP I)
   29. Interphal. joint I (IPH)
   30. Distal phalanx I (PD I)

Terminology of the foot; shaded
areas on skeletal parts are
visible, and palpable under the skin.

B. First ray of the foot
   DP   distal phalanx
   PP   proximal phalanx
   MT   interphalangeal joint
   IPH   big toe (hallux)
   MTP   metatarsophalangeal joint
   TMT   tarsometatarsal joint

C. Second to fifth ray
   of the foot
   DP   distal phalanx
   MP   middle phalanx
   PP   proximal phalanx
   MT   metatarsal
   DIP   distal interphalang. joint
   PIP   prox. interphal. joint
   MTP   metatarsophalang. joint
   TMT   tarsometatarsal joint

D. a-a   Axis of foot (through
          second metatarsal and
          second toe)

   I   big toe (first toe)
   II   second toe
   III   third toe
   IV   fourth toe
   V   fifth toe

E. 1.   tarsal joints
   2.   talonavicular joint
   3.   talocrural joint (upper
        ankle joint)
   4.   talocalcaneal joint (sub-
        talar or lower ankle
        joint)

Abbreviations:

MT	metatarsal bone	TMT	tarsometatarsal joint	IPH	interphalangeal joint I
PP	proximal phalanx	MTP	metatarsophalangeal joint	PAP	forefoot
MP	middle phalanx	PIP	proximal interphalangeal joint	PMP	midfoot
DP	distal phalanx	DIP	distal interphalangeal joint	PPP	hindfoot

Measuring points and construction line redrawn from; Lanz, Wachsmuth,
Praktische Anatomie, Bein und Statik, Berlin, Verlag Julius Springer, 1938.

TERMINOLOGIA PEDIS

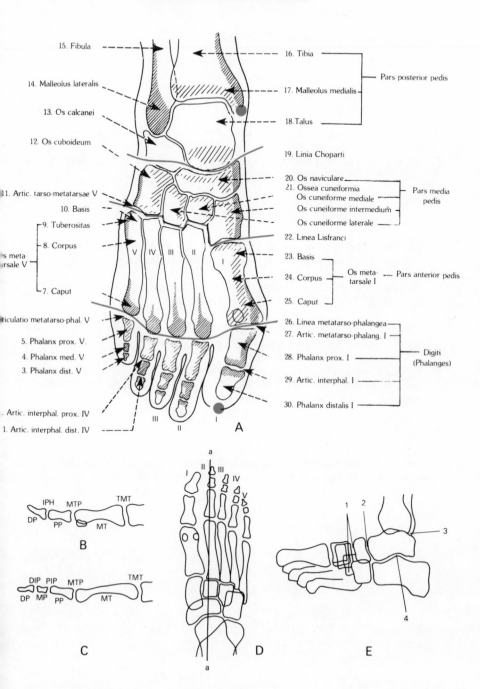

15. Fibula

14. Malleolus lateralis

13. Os calcanei

12. Os cuboideum

11. Artic. tarso-metatarsae V

10. Basis

9. Tuberositas

8. Corpus

Os meta-
tarsale V

7. Caput

Articulatio metatarso-phal. V

5. Phalanx prox. V.

4. Phalanx med. V

3. Phalanx dist. V

. Artic. interphal. prox. IV

1. Artic. interphal. dist. IV

16. Tibia

17. Malleolus medialis

Pars posterior pedis

18. Talus

19. Linia Choparti

20. Os naviculare

21. Ossea cuneiformia
    Os cuneiforme mediale
    Os cuneiforme intermedium
    Os cuneiforme laterale

Pars media
pedis

22. Linea Lisfranci

23. Basis

24. Corpus — Os meta-
tarsale I — Pars anterior pedis

25. Caput

26. Linea metatarso-phalangea

27. Artic. metatarso-phalang. I

28. Phalanx prox. I

Digiti
(Phalanges)

29. Artic. interphal. I

30. Phalanx distalis I

A

IPH   MTP   TMT
DP   PP   MT

B

DIP PIP   MTP   TMT
DP MP PP   MT

C

a

I   II   III
         IV
           V

D

a

1   2
          3

4

E

MEASUREMENTS OF THE FOOT

MEASUREMENTS OF THE FOOT

1. The long axis of the foot extends through to the middle of the heel, second metatarsal and second toe.

2. Pes Metatarsus Valgus (Abductus) 35^0 SFTR-Recording: T:35-0.

3. Pes Metatarsus Varus (Adductus) 40^0 SFTR-Recording: T:0-40.

4. Extension and flexion of the great toe at the metatarsophalangeal joint (MTP I). SFTR-Recording: S:70-0-45.

5. Hallux valgus angle between long axis of first metatarsal (MT I) and proximal phalanx (PP I) is 50^0. SFTR-Recording: T:50-0.

6. Digitus quintus varus angle between long axis of fifth metatarsal (MT V), and proximal phalanx (PP V), is 45^0. SFTR-Recording: T:0-45

7. Extension and flexion at the metatarsophalangeal joints of second to fifth toes (MTP II-V). SFTR-Recording: S:40-0-35

8. Extension and flexion at the proximal interphalangeal joint of second to fifth toes (PIP II-V). SFTR-Recording: S:0-0-40.

9. Extension and flexion at the distal interphalangeal joints of second to fifth toes (DIP II-V). In Figure 9, there is (pathological) hyperextension of 30^0 present. SFTR-Recording: S:30-0-55.

Remarks:
    Usually limitations of motion of toes is only estimated and may be expressed in two ways, "the motion of a given toe is 2/3, 1/2, or 1/3 of normal", or "the motion of a given toe is 1/3, 1/2, or 2/3 restricted".

PES
(MENSURAE PEDIS)

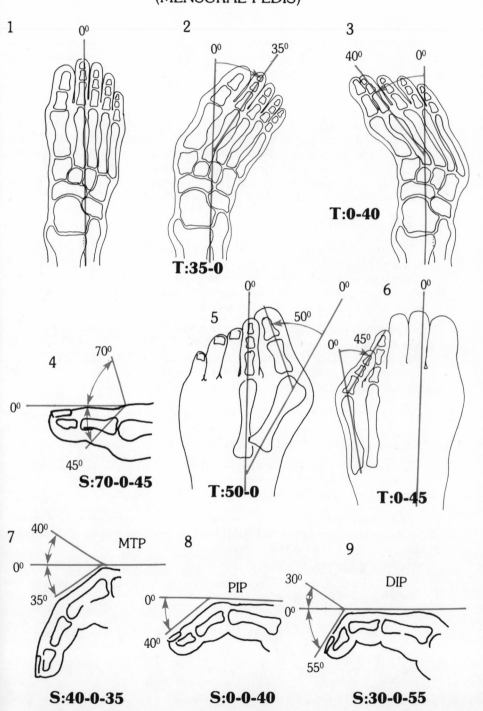

1   0°

2   0°   35°
T:35-0

3   40°   0°
T:0-40

4   70°
0°
45°
S:70-0-45

5   0°   0°   50°
T:50-0

6   0°   0°   45°
T:0-45

7   40°   MTP
0°
35°
S:40-0-35

8   PIP
0°
40°
S:0-0-40

9   30°   DIP
0°
55°
S:30-0-55

THE PLURIMETER

DESCRIPTION

When treating limitations of joint movements, one of the important criteria for assessment of the efficiency of therapy is the evaluation of changes of joint movements. For over one hundred years, the instrument used was a two-armed goniometer. It had advantages but also many disadvantages which will be described later.

With the PLURIMETER SYSTEM, Dr. Rippstein created a measuring instrument of superb qualities. It provides not only increased speed and accuracy, but also allows much easier reading of the measurements. It also allows measurements that were not possible with the conventional goniometers. This includes accurate measurements of the spine, supination, pronation of the forearm and the foot, and tibial torsion among others.

HISTORICAL ASPECTS

The first goniometer of the new measuring instruments was the Hydro-Goniometer, a hydraulic inclinometer. It was awarded the Gold Medal in 1967 at the International Inventors Fair, in Brussels, Belgium. Approximately 174,000 units were produced by the pharmacalogical company Geigy, in Switzerland, and distributed as a promotion item to physicians all over the world.

During the next 22 years of continuous research, Dr. Rippstein perfected the system which finally evolved into the PLURIMETER device and MODULAR MEASURING SYSTEM. In 1987, at the International Inventors Fair in Basel, Switzerland, the system was awarded a gold medal, and Dr. Rippstein received special recognition for the best results of long-term research.

With the PLURIMETER, Dr. Rippstein developed a superb precision measuring device. It is especially suited for application in the NEUTRAL-ZERO-MEASURING and SFTR-RECORDING methods.

The combination of these methods with the PLURIMETER instrumentation provides an ideal and truly international standardized system for measuring and documentation of joint motion.

The accuracy, reproducibility, speed and ease of application, and brevity and clarity of documentation will appeal not only to researchers and disability evaluators, but also to the busy clinician.

1. The PLURIMETER
2. The PLURI-CAL is the Plurimeter attached to a caliper as part of the *MODULAR SYSTEM*

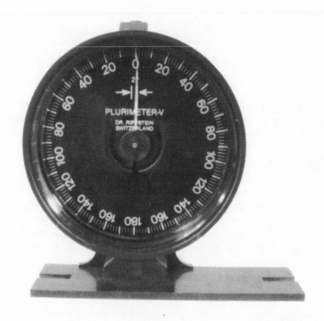

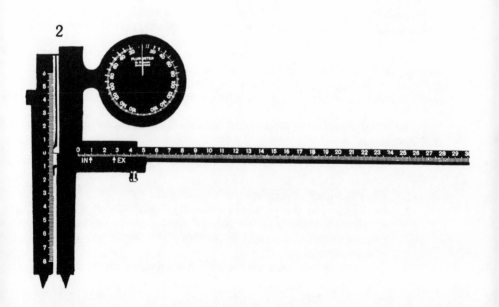

THE PLURIMETER

PRINCIPLE OF FUNCTION

The Plurimeter consists of a container with a freely moving needle that is counterweighted to keep it in a vertical position. The housing is filled with a special oil, which lubricates the bearing of the axis and dampens the oscillations of the needle-indicator when the instrument is rotated. The face of the dial with the degrees is large and allows easy and clear readings. The housing can be rotated 360^0. It locks automatically at 90^0 intervals allowing easy determination of a horizontal or vertical position. Application and reading errors are therefore practically eliminated.

The combination of the Plurimeter with special attachments described in the appropriate sections of this book, allows additional accurate measurements. They include measurements of eversion and inversion of the hindfoot and midfoot, which are of great importance to the pediatric orthopedic surgeon, the supination and pronation of the forearm, and tibial torsion. Heights of the rib hump or lumbar bulge in clinical assessment of rotational scoliosis, and x-ray measurements of leg shortening and external and internal diameters of prosthetic sockets and orthotic devices can also be measured easily.

GENERAL APPLICATION

The Plurimeter has to be applied in a vertical position to allow free movement of the needle-indicator. The subject or measured limb has to be positioned accordingly.

The base of the Plurimeter substitutes for the conventional stationary and movable arms and has to be held steadily on the moving part of the body or limb.

The Plurimeter is held between the index and middle finger of one hand, leaving the thumb, ring and little fingers of the same hand to stabilize the instrument on the moving part of the body while the other hand of the examiner is free for stabilization of the body or guidance of the motion.

The advantages of the system and detailed application are described in the following pages.

1. The PLURIMETER is held with one hand.
2. The PLURIMETER is stabilized on the forehead with one hand, to measure rotation of the cervical spine.
3. The rotating dial shows clear numbers, the needle-indicator is always vertical.
4. Changes of inclination of the base are reflected on the dial in degrees.

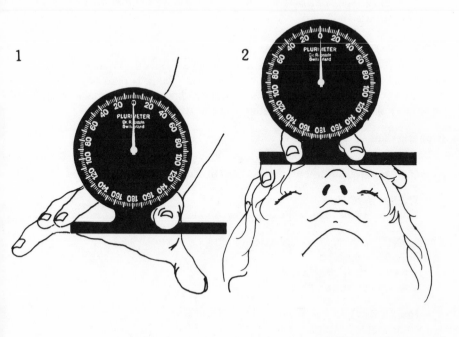

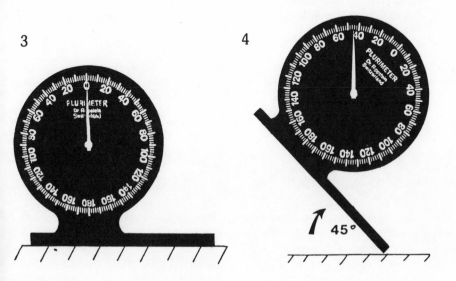

45°

65

ADVANTAGES OF THE PLURIMETER

The advantages of the Pluri-V in comparison with conventional two- armed goniometers are multiple:

Large clear dial:

The dial of the goniometer is large and clear (Figure 2). There is only one row of numbers, which are large and easy to read. There is only one arrow -- the indicator -- so that instant and accurate readings of the measurements are assured. False or ambiguous readings are virtually impossible.

Rotating dial:

The zero position can be easily set it locks in a vertical or horizontal position, allowing easy measurements in the Neutral-Zero Measuring Method.

1. *ANKLE JOINT*
    Ankle in 10^0 of plantar flexion position.

2. *CONVENTIONAL GONIOMETER*
    Confusing dial
    Numbers difficult to read
    Reading errors possible

3. *PLURIMETER*
    Clear dial
    Only one line of numbers
    Only one movable vector
    Big numbers, easy to read
    No reading errors

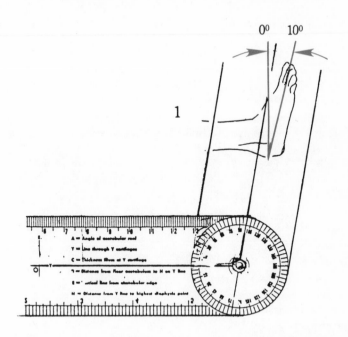

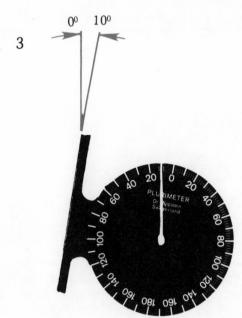

ADVANTAGES OF THE PLURIMETER

SIMPLICITY OF APPLICATION

1. Only two fingers are required to hold the Plurimeter.
    The same hand that holds the Plurimeter, guides motion.
    The other hand remains free for palpation, stabilization or passive guidance of motion of the measured part.

2. The hand that holds the Plurimeter guides the head through extension and flexion. The other hand stabilizes the shoulder.

3. A-A -- notches for easy grip between index and middle fingers.

ACCURACY

Vertical and Neutral-Zero Starting Position are automatically indicated.

4. *CONVENTIONAL GONIOMETER*

    Vertical and Neutral-0-Starting Position are estimated
    Lack of accuracy
    There is no free hand to support the arm

5. *PLURIMETER*

    Vertical and Neutral-0-Starting Position are automatically indicated.
    One hand is free to support the arm.

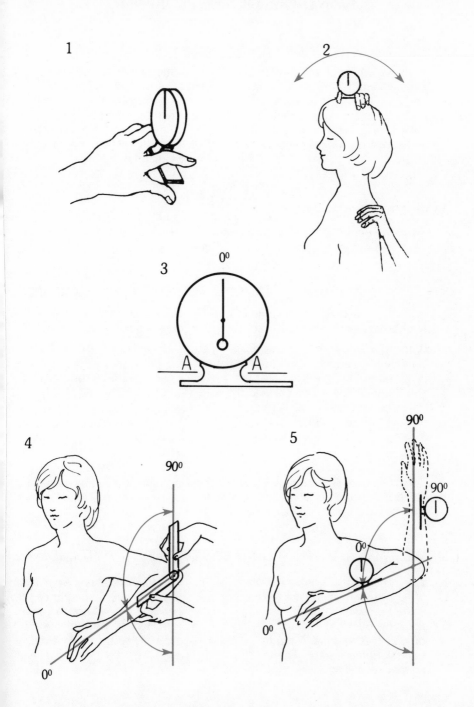

ADVANTAGES OF THE PLURIMETER

MEASURING OF SCOLIOSIS ANGLE IN X-RAYS

1. With the conventional goniometer supplementary lines must be drawn on X-ray films (not desirable). Lines are often poorly visible on dark X-rays. Several sources of measuring errors are encountered

2. With the Plurimeter no structured lines are needed on X-ray film. Dial is turned to 0⁰ in "A" position then the Plurimeter moved to "B" position and Cobbs Scoliosis angle read directly in an exact and simple manner.

NEW MEASURING POSSIBILITIES

Measurements of positionings and motion that could not be taken until now, can be measured in a simple, precise and quick manner.

MEASURING OF KYPHOSIS ANGLE

3. With the conventional goniometer kyphosis angle is not measurable.

4. With the Plurimeter kyphosis angle is easily measurable. The Plurimeter is placed at "A", the dial set at 0⁰ and the instrument repositioned to "B". The kyphosis angle is read directly on the dial (40⁰).

MOTION OF THORACIC SPINE

5. Cannot be measured with the conventional goniometer.

6. Can be easily measured with the Plurimeter. The thoracic spine is first measured with the person in prone position on the table, then measured again in the sphinx position. The variations indicates motion in degrees.

To measure maximum mobility of the thoracic spine, the kyphosis angle is measured in standing position and then in the sphinx position. The difference indicates passive motion in degrees.

MEASUREMENTS WITH APPLICATIONS DISTANT FROM THE JOINT

7. The *conventional goniometer* has to be placed over the approximate center of rotation and the arms over the long axis of joint components. Measurements are inaccurate. There is poor reproducibility.

8. The *Plurimeter can be placed distant from the center of rotation* and it need not to be determined. Measurements are accurate with excellent reproducibility.

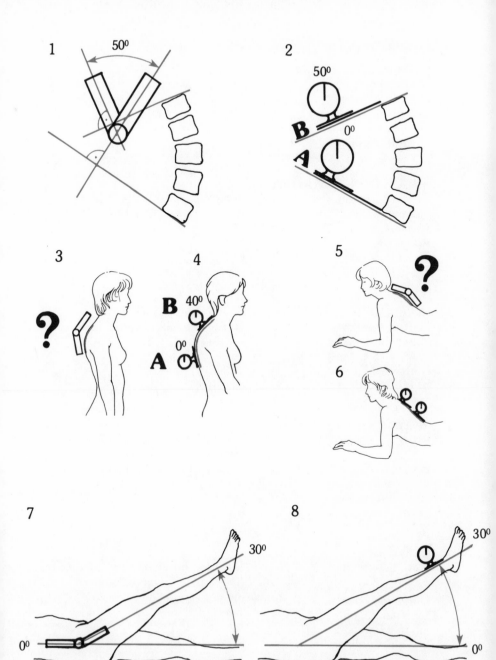

1

50⁰

2

50⁰

B

0⁰

A

3

?

4

B 40⁰

A 0⁰

5

?

6

7

30⁰

0⁰

8

30⁰

0⁰

71

PLURIMETER-SHOULDER

MEASUREMENTS OF THE SHOULDER

1. EXTENSION-FLEXION
   Starting position: anatomical position (arm at side of body)
   Plurimeter base: on long axis of arm, dial at 0^0
   Extension: 40^0
   Flexion: 170^0
   SFTR-Recording: S:40-0-170

2. ABDUCTION-ADDUCTION
   Starting position: anatomical position (arm at side of body)
   Plurimeter base: on long axis of arm, dial at 0^0
   Abduction: 180^0
   Adduction: 45^0
   SFTR-Recording: F:180-0-45

3. HORIZONTAL EXTENSION-HORIZONTAL FLEXION
   Starting position: supine (shoulder beyond table)
   Plurimeter base   on long axis of arm, dial at 0^0
   Horizontal Extension: 20^0
   Horizontal Flexion: 135^0
   SFTR-Recording: T:20-0-135

4. ROTATION
   Starting position: standing or supine. Arm in 90^0 abduction, elbow 90^0 flexion
   Plurimeter base: on axis of forearm, dial 0^0
   External Rotation: 90^0
   Internal Rotation: 80^0
   SFTR-Recording: R(F90):90-0-80 or R:90-0-80 (standard)

5. ROTATION
   Starting position: side-lying position, arm at side of body, (F0), elbow flexed to 90^0
   Plurimeter base: on axis of forearm
   External Rotation: 45^0
   Internal Rotation: 40^0
   SFTR-Recording: R(Fo):45-0-40

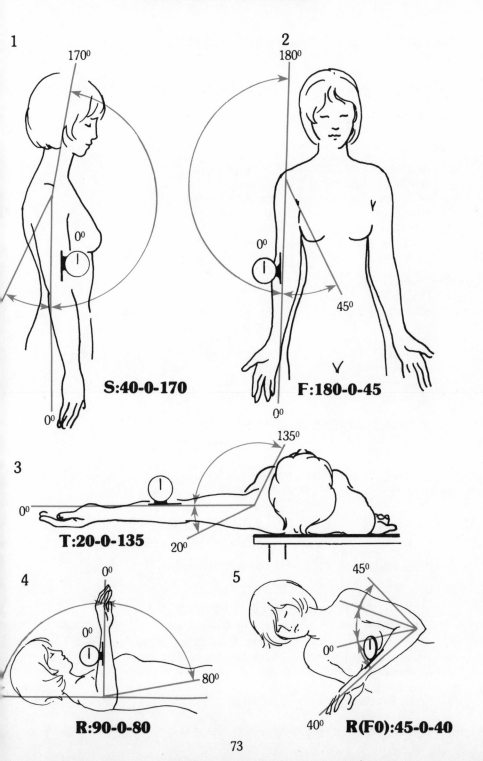

1 170° 0° 0° **S:40-0-170**

2 180° 0° 45° 0° **F:180-0-45**

3 135° 0° 20° **T:20-0-135**

4 0° 0° 80° **R:90-0-80**

5 45° 0° 40° **R(F0):45-0-40**

PLURIMETER-SHOULDER GIRDLE, ELBOW, FOREARM

MEASUREMENTS OF THE SHOULDER GIRDLE
1. ELEVATION-DEPRESSION

Starting position:	standing
Plurimeter base:	horizontal on shoulder (acromion-clavicle)
Elevation:	35^0
Depression:	20^0
SFTR-Recording:	F:35-0-20

2. RETRACTION-PROTRACTION (of scapula)

Starting position:	supine
Plurimeter base	horizontal on shoulder
Retraction:	10^0
Protraction:	20^0
SFTR-Recording:	T:10-0-20

MEASUREMENTS OF THE ELBOW
3. FLEXION

Starting position:	elbow extended in continuation of long axis of arm
Plurimeter base:	Placed on forearm.
Extension	usually 0^0 physiological in some individuals.
Hyperextension:	10^0
Flexion:	135^0
SFTR-Recording:	S:10-0-135

4. FLEXION DEFORMITY OF THE ELBOW

Starting position:	same as in #3. Elbow cannot be extended
Plurimeter base:	first placed on long axis of arm or its extension arc is set at 0^0, the base is repositioned on forearm. The dial shows actual starting position of 50^0
Flexion deformity:	50^0
Total flexion:	to 90^0
SFTR-Recording:	S:0-50-90

5. SUPINATION-PRONATION OF FOREARM

Starting position:	hand in S plane, arm close to the body elbow flexed at 90^0, do not lift elbow
Plurimeter base:	on volar side of the wrist
Supination:	90^0
Pronation:	80^0
SFTR-Recording:	R:90-0-80

ARTICULATIONES CINGULI MEMBRI SUPERIORIS, ART. CUBITI ET RADIO-ULNARIS PROX. ET DIST.

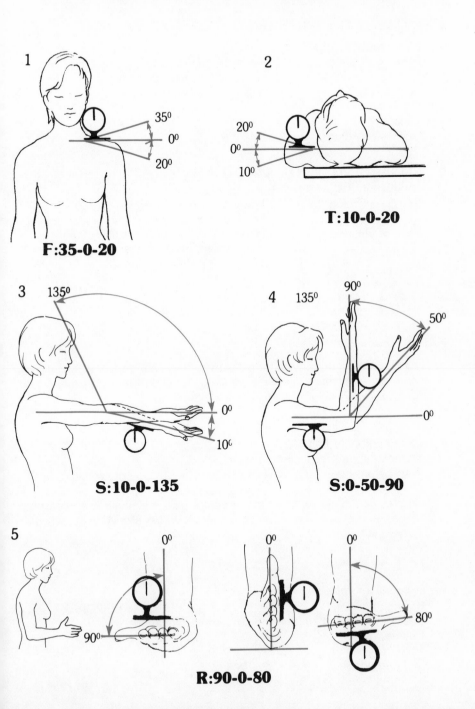

1

35⁰
0⁰
20⁰

F:35-0-20

2

20⁰
0⁰
10⁰

T:10-0-20

3   135⁰

0⁰
10⁰

S:10-0-135

4   135⁰   90⁰

50⁰

0⁰

S:0-50-90

5   0⁰   0⁰   0⁰

90⁰

80⁰

R:90-0-80

PLURIMETER-WRIST AND HAND

MEASUREMENTS OF THE WRIST

1. EXTENSION-FLEXION

Starting Position	forearm horizontal and pronated with wrist in neutral position
Base of Plurimeter	aligned with metacarpal III
Extension	60⁰
Flexion	40⁰
SFTR-Recording	S:60-0-40

Extension 60^0
Flexion 40^0

2. RADIAL DEVIATION-ULNAR DEVIATION
(Abduction-Adduction)

Starting position	forearm in neutral rotation (mid position between supination and pronation).
Base of Plurimeter	Hand in Neutral-Zero position aligned with metacarpal III and extended digit. Forearm must be stabilized.
Radial deviation	35^0
Ulnar deviation	30^0
SFTR-Recording	F:35-0-30

HAND

The Plurimeter can be used for measurements of hand and finger joints, but it is more convenient to use a specially designed finger goniometer, the PLURI-DIG (Digital Plurimeter), described later.

3. EXTENSION-FLEXION
Metacarpophalangeal joints II-V (MCP)

Starting position	forearm in neutral position, pronated, hand in neutral position
Base of Plurimeter	on dorsum of proximal phalanx of measured digit. Finger extended aligned with metacarpals
Extension	20^0
Flexion	80^0
SFTR-Recording	S:20-0-80

4. Proximal interphalangeal joint II-V (PIP)

Starting position	same as above but proximal phalanx stabilized
Base of Plurimeter	on dorsum of middle phalanx
Extension	20^0
Flexion	95^0
SFTR-Recording	S:20-0-95

ARTICULATIO RADIOULNARIS DISTALIS
ARTICULATIO RADIOCARPEA ET MANUS

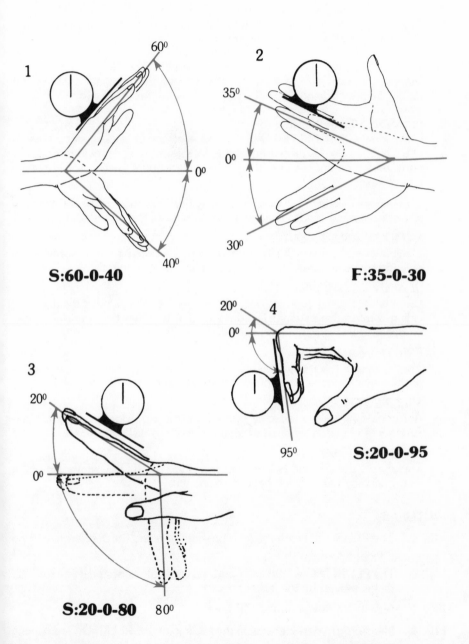

1

60^0

0^0

40^0

S:60-0-40

2

35^0

0^0

30^0

F:35-0-30

3

20^0

0^0

S:20-0-80 80^0

4

20^0

0^0

95^0

S:20-0-95

PLURIMETER − DIGITS
THE PLURI · DIG

This single hand operated finger goniometer, has the following advantages.

1. *ONLY ONE HAND IS NEEDED TO OPERATE THE INSTRUMENT*
    The PLURI-DIG is a single hand operating goniometer. The other hand of the examiner is free to move the joint.

    This has been achieved by enlarging the handle 12 cm. long ergonomically shaped grip, which is comfortably held between the examiner's thumb and middle fingers, freeing the index finger to move the rotation dial.

2. *PRECISE MEASUREMENTS*
    Measuring with the PLURI-DIG is more accurate because hyperextension of a digit may also be measured on the dorsal side, which provides a straight bony reference line, wheras the palmar side with its uneven soft tissue, is less reliable.

    This feature has been achieved by moving the 0^0 position on the dial from the straight base-line to 40^0; changing the position of the instrument.

3. *RAPID MEASUREMENT*
    Eliminations of shifting the instrument from the dorsal to the volar side not only improves accuracy but also speeds up measurements.

4. *READING COMFORT*
    Large white figures contrast well with the black background of the dial, providing comfortable reading. The division of 5^0 to 5^0 has been carefully chosen because this is much easier to read than the 1^0 to 1^0 division.

5. *FRICTION ADAPTER*
    The friction of the moving dial can be adapted to the personal preference of the investigator by loosening or tighting the friction screw.

6. *MILLIMETER SCALE*
    A 10 cm. long millimeter-scale printed on the grip, allows functional measurements of distances such as fingertip to palm distances easily.

7. *RIGHT-LEFT-HANDED*
    The shape, the dial and two indicators of the PLURI-DIG allows use of the instrument by right- or left-handed examiners.

PICTURES

FIG. 1. The PLURI-DIG with the long baseline grip and the 0^0 reference being moved 40^0 upwards.

FIG. 2. The PLURI-DIG is held and operated with only one hand. (The rotation dial is moved by the index finger.)

FIG. 3. Measuring flexion in the PIP joint.

FIG. 4. Measuring hyperextension in the MCP joint, the PLURI-DIG remaining on the dorsal side of the finger.

MENSURAE DIGITORUM

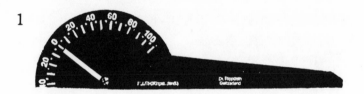

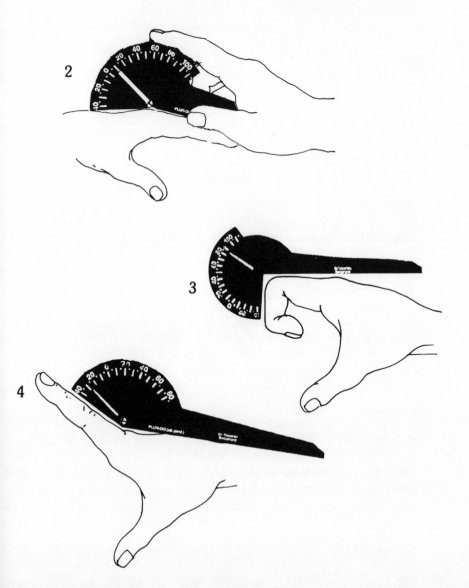

PLURIMETER-CERVICAL AND THORACIC SPINE

MEASUREMENTS OF THE CERVICAL SPINE

1. EXTENSION-FLEXION
Starting position:	sitting or standing
Extension:	45^0
Flexion:	65^0
SFTR-Recording:	S:45-0-65

2. LATERAL BENDING
Starting position:	sitting or standing
Left:	55^0
Right:	45^0
SFTR-Recording:	F:55-0-45

3. ROTATION
Starting position:	supine
Left:	75^0
Right:	70^0
SFTR-Recording:	R:75-0-70

MEASUREMENTS OF THORACIC SPINE

4. KYPHOSIS
Starting position: standing

The Plurimeter is placed on the lower part of the kyphosis and the dial set on 0^0; the instrument is then repositioned to the upper part of the kyphosis. The angle is read directly at the dial. Kyphosis of 50^0 is recorded S:0-50.

5. MOBILITY OF THORACIC SPINE
The patient is placed in a sphinx position and the application of the Plurimeter repeated as in 4 (standing or prone). The angle of kyphosis is read. The difference between the former and latter angle indicates mobility expressed in degrees. The kyphosis angle in the sphinx position of 30^0 is recorded S:0-30. The mobility of the thoracic spine is thus 20^0.
SFTR Recording: S:0-30-50.

6,7,8. ROTATION
The pelvis is stabilized on the table, the trunk supported and rotated to the left and to the right. The Plurimeter is held over the sternum.
SFTR Recording: R:45-0-45

The rotation to the left is recorded first (to the *left* of 0), and to the right last (to the *right* of 0).

COLUMNA VERTEBRALIS CERVICALIS ET THORACALIS

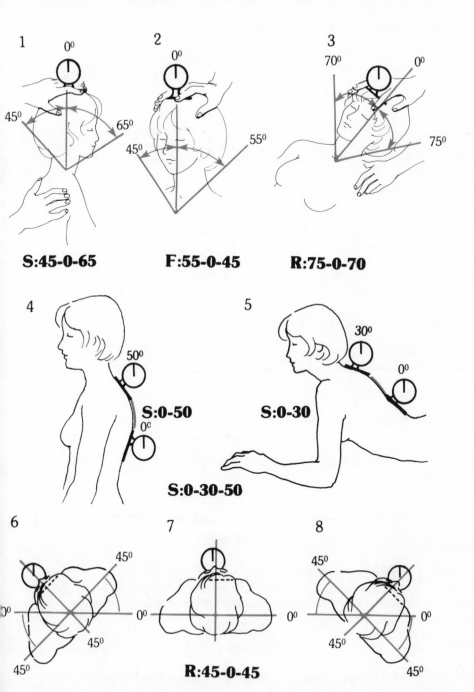

1

0^0

45^0 65^0

S:45-0-65

2

0^0

45^0 55^0

F:55-0-45

3

70^0 0^0

75^0

R:75-0-70

4

50^0

S:0-50

0^c

S:0-30-50

5

30^0

0^0

S:0-30

6

45^0

0^0

45^0

45^0

7

0^0

R:45-0-45

8

45^0

0^0

45^0

45^0

PLURIMETER-LUMBAR SPINE

MEASUREMENTS OF LUMBAR SPINE

1. *EXTENSION:*
   The plurimeter is placed on the upper part of the lumbar spine, the dial set at $0°$, the spine extended, and the extension angle of $30°$ read directly. Extension   S:30-0-0.

2. *FLEXION:*
   Bending forward is a combined flexion of the hips, pelvic tilt and the flexion of the lumbar spine .The flexion of the lumbar spine alone will be obtained by the subtraction of the hip-flexion and pelvic tilt from the total movement.

2A. Total movement:
   (Flexion of the hip, pelvic tilt and flexion of the lumbar spine).

   a. Place the Plurimeter on the upper part of the lumbar spine (L1), and set the dial at $0°$.

   b. Bend forward and read the angle of the combined motion at $95°$. S:0-0-95

2B. Flexion of hips and pelvic tilt.

   a. Place the Plurimeter on the sacrum and set the dial at $0°$.

   b. Bend foreward and read the angle at $45°$. S:0-0-45

   A Combined lumbar spine, pelvic tilt and hip flexion: $95°$
             pelvic tilt and hip flexion: $\underline{45°}$

   - B Flexion of the lumbar spine proper is: $50°$

   SFTR: S:0-0- $50°$

   Total motion of the lumbar spine with extension of $30°$ and flexion of $50°$ is recorded: **S:30-0-50**

3. *LATERAL BENDING*
   The plurimeter is placed with the base horizontal at the L1 level and the dial set at $0°$. Lateral bending to the left $50°$. Lateral bending to the right $35°$.

   F:50-0-35

4. Cobb's scoliosis angle (levo-scoliosis-convexity on left side).

COLUMNA VERTEBRALIS LUMBALIS

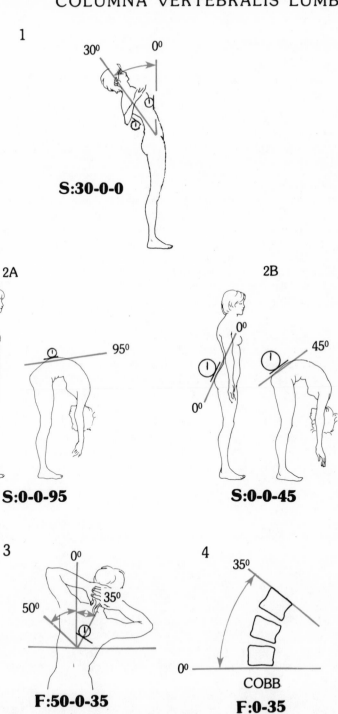

1

30⁰   0⁰

S:30-0-0

2A

0⁰   95⁰

S:0-0-95

2B

0⁰   45⁰
0⁰

S:0-0-45

3

0⁰
50⁰   35⁰

F:50-0-35

4

35⁰
0⁰
COBB

F:0-35

PLURIMETER-HIP

MEASUREMENTS OF THE HIP

1. *EXTENSION* (S-Plane)
   Extension of the hip is measured in the prone position with the opposite hip flexed over the edge of the table. It is used only for the evaluation of passive motion of the hip. One hand stabilizes the pelvis to minimize the movements of the pelvis and of the lumbar spine. The Plurimeter is placed parallel to the long axis of the thigh or the leg (over the popliteal fossa or Achilles tendon with the knee extended). SFTR recording is: S:15-0-0. There is no physiological extension of the hip joint proper.

2. *FLEXION* (S-Plane)
   Flexion of the hip is measured in the supine position. The opposite hip is extended. Pelvis and spine must be immobilized. The Thomas maneuver is used to detect hip flexion contracture. One hand stabilizes the pelvis to avoid movements of the lumbar spine. The Plurimeter is placed over the distal thigh. Hip flexion measures 130^0. Hip (extension and flexion) is recorded as S:15-0-130. (Pictures 1 and 2.)
   The combined flexion of the hip and lumbar spine with hip flexion contracture of 30^0 is recorded as: S:0-30-130.

3. *ABDUCTION-ADDUCTION* (F-Plane)
   Measurements of abduction and adduction of the hip with the Plurimeter must be done in a side-lying position. The Plurimeter is placed parallel to the long axis of the thigh or leg. The abduction is 45^0, the adduction is 30^0. Important: pelvis must be immobilized. SFTR Recording: F:45-0-30

4. *HORIZONTAL ABDUCTION-HORIZONTAL ADDUCTION* (T-Plane)
   Horizontal abduction and adduction is measured in the supine position with the hips flexed 90^0. The Plurimeter is applied on the lateral aspect of the thigh.

   Horizontal abduction is 45^0, horizontal adduction is 30^0.
   SFTR Recording: T:45-0-30

ARTICULATIO COXAE

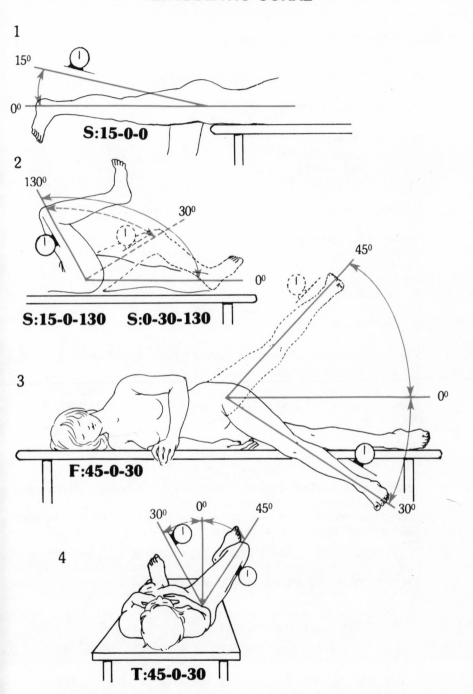

1

15⁰

0⁰

S:15-0-0

2

130⁰

30⁰

0⁰

S:15-0-130 **S:0-30-130**

45⁰

0⁰

3

F:45-0-30

30⁰

4

30⁰ 0⁰ 45⁰

T:45-0-30

PLURIMETER-HIP ROTATION

MEASUREMENTS OF HIP ROTATION

1-3. Hip rotation can be measured in various positions.
Rotation in prone position.
Hip is extended and the knee flexed 90^0.
The Plurimeter is applied parallel to the tibial crest
which serves as vector of motion.

External Rotation: 60^0 (1)
Neutral-Zero Starting Position: 0^0 (2)
Internal Rotation: 35^0 (3)

4. Rotation in sitting position.
Hip and knee in 90^0 flexion.
Plurimeter on lateral leg.
SFTR-Recording: R(Hip S90, Knee S90):60-0-30 *

5. Rotation in supine position.
Hip extended knee in 90^0 flexion.
The opposite hip flexed, Plurimeter on lateral leg.
SFTR-Recording: R(S0, Knee S90):60-0-30

6. Rotation in supine position in subjects with ankylosis of knee in extension and the hip extended:

The Plurimeter is applied on the long axis of the foot which serves as vector of motion. Rotation of foot, knee and hip has to be performed as a unit.

SFTR-Recording: R(S0, Knee S0):45-0-30

* If the starting position requires positioning of the extremity different than the neutral position, than indication of the positioning is recorded in parentheses after indication of motion. In picture 4, measuring of the hip, the hip is measured with the hip flexed 90^0 and the knee flexed 90^0.

In the short recording, names of the joints (hip, knee etc.), can be omitted when we agree that position of the proximal joint is recorded (hip), first and the position of the distal joint (knee), second. R(S90, S90):60-0-30.

ARTICULATIO COXAE

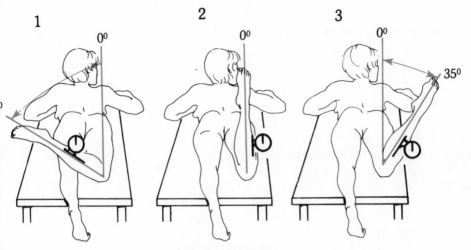

R(S0):60-0-35

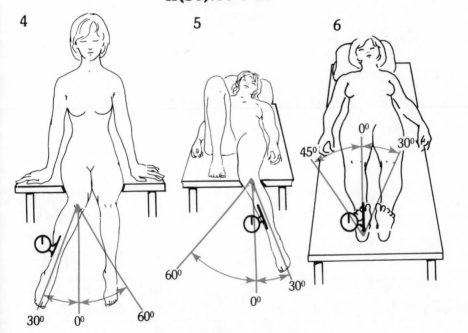

R(S0, S90):60-0-30

R(S90, S90):60-0-30

R(S0, S0):45-0-30

PLURIMETER-HIP AND AMPUTATIONS

MEASUREMENTS OF THE HIP

SPECIAL CONSIDERATIONS.

1. *STRAIGHT LEG RAISING   (LASEQUE)*
   Patient is in supine position.
   The Plurimeter is placed over the distal tibia at 0^0, the straight leg raised and the angle of hip flexion read directly on the dial.
   Recording: SLR S:0-80.

2. *QUADRICEPS TIGHTNESS* (ELY test):
   Patient is in prone position.
   The Plurimeter is placed over the Achilles tendon at 0^0.
   The knee flexed maximally and the angle read directly on the dial. When flexing the knee do not allow hip flexion.
   Recording: ELY S:0-110.

3. *ANKYLOSIS OF THE HIP AT 30^0*
   The Thomas maneuver is used to arrest the lumbar spine and make the true angle of the hip flexion apparent.
   The position of the ankylotic hip is measured.
   Recording: S:0-30.

ABOVE-KNEE AMPUTATION STUMP

4. Measuring adduction (inclination) of the lateral wall of 5^0.

5. Measuring hip flexion (initial flexion is 10^0).

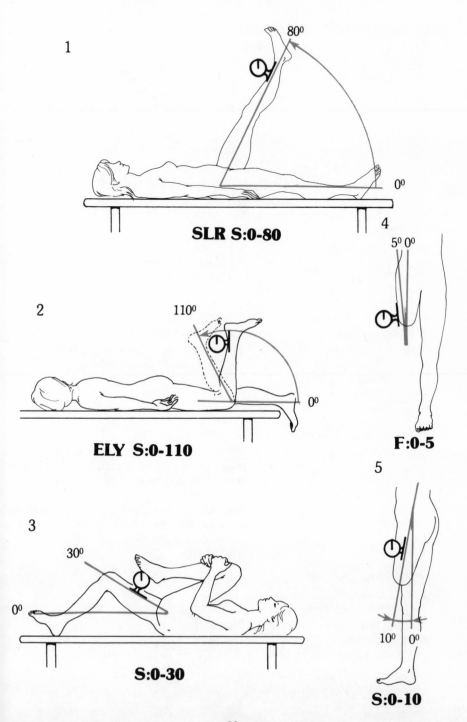

1

SLR S:0-80

2

ELY S:0-110

3

S:0-30

4

F:0-5

5

S:0-10

PLURIMETER-ANKLE

MEASUREMENTS OF THE ANKLE
TALO-CRURAL (Upper Ankle) Joint

1. **WEIGHTBEARING EXTENSION (Dorsiflexion)**

Starting position:	Standing, feet parallel, avoid external rotation of leg and heel valgus
Base of Plurimeter:	Base is placed over the tibia
Extension:	30^0
Flexion:	0^0
SFTR-Recording:	S:30-0-0.

2. **WEIGHTBEARING FLEXION (Plantar flexion)**

   Same as above. Only partial weightbearing can be applied to the ankle in standing position with measured ankle moved forward, or sitting with knees slightly bent.

Starting position:	Standing or sitting.
Plurimeter base:	Placed over tibia.
SFTR-Recording:	S:0-0-40

3. **NON-WEIGHTBEARING EXTENSION-FLEXION**

Starting position:	Supine, leg supported.
Base of Plurimeter:	Base is pressed against a small board which is placed over sole of foot.
Extension (dorsiflexion):	15^0
Plantar flexion:	45^0
SFTR-Recording:	S:15-0-45

4. **NON-WEIGHTBEARING ALTERNATE POSITION**

Starting position:	When heel cords are tight, the subject may kneel on a table with hips and knees flexed 90^0 and foot-ankle free beyond the edge of the table. The patient may also be in prone position with the knee flexed 90^0. The legs must be stabilized during measurements.
Extension:	20^0
Flexion:	45^0
SFTR-Recording:	S:20-0-45

TALO-CALCANEAL (Lower Ankle) Joint.

5. **VALGUS OF HEELS**

Starting position:	Standing
Base of Plurimeter:	Parallel to calcaneal axis.
SFTR-Recording:	FC:20-0

6. **VARUS OF HEELS**

   Same as above but heels in varus position.

SFTR-Recording:	FC:0-15

ARTICULATIO TALO-CRURALIS
ET TALO CALCANEI

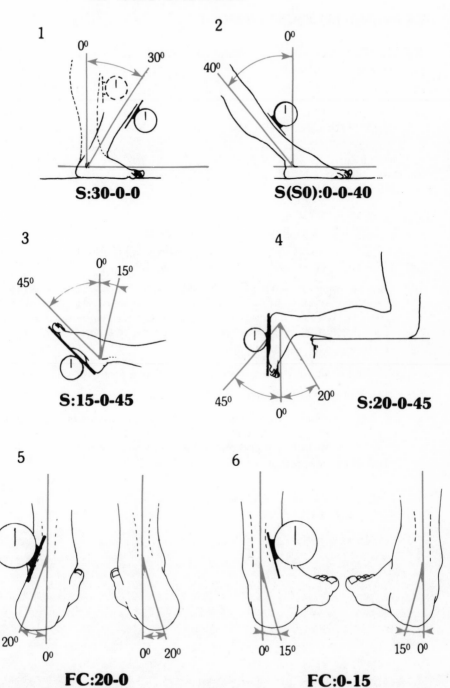

1

0⁰

30⁰

S:30-0-0

2

0⁰

40⁰

S(S0):0-0-40

3

0⁰ 15⁰

45⁰

S:15-0-45

4

45⁰ 20⁰

0⁰

S:20-0-45

5

20⁰

0⁰ 0⁰ 20⁰

FC:20-0

6

0⁰ 15⁰ 15⁰ 0⁰

FC:0-15

PLURIMETER-FOOT

MEASUREMENTS OF THE HINDFOOT

JOINTS: Talo-calcaneal, Talo-calcaeo navicular (lower ankle joint)

Eversion - Inversion of hindfoot PP (pars posterior)
Position: prone with knee flexed 90^0; upper ankle joint and leg stabilized.

1,2. Technique of application of the Plurimeter and stabilization of the talocrural (upper ankle) joint of the leg.
3. Eversion of hindfoot
4. Neutral-Zero
5. Inversion of hindfoot
   SFTR-Recording: FPP:10-0-10

MEASUREMENTS OF THE MIDFOOT
Eversion and Inversion of midfoot, PM (pars media)

Joints: Talo-calcaneo-navicular, Calcaneo-cuboid (CHOPART),
Cuneo-cuboid, Intercuneiform, Cuneo-navicular joints.

6. Position same as above. The Plurimeter with attachment plate is placed over the midfoot distal to the talo-calcaneo-navicular and calcaneo-cuboid joints (CHOPART). The heel and leg are stabilized with the other hand. Dial is set at 0^0 and the midfoot everted and inverted.

   SFTR-Recording: FPM:10-0-10

   Alternate Position: leg and knee lateral on table, foot over edge of table.

7. The Plurimeter attachment for ankle and foot measurements.

   The foot plate allows more precise measurements
   of extension - flexion of the ankle, eversion - inversion
   of the hindfoot and midfoot and supination - pronation
   of the forefoot.

ARTICULATIONES PEDIS
(PARS POSTERIOR ET PARS MEDIA)

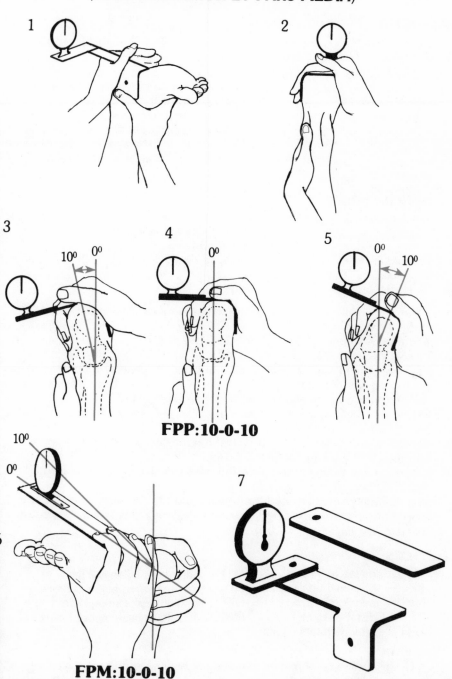

FPP:10-0-10

FPM:10-0-10

PLURIMETER-FOOT

FOREFOOT

Joints: Cuneiforme I-metatarsal I, Cunei-metatarsals II-III, Cuboid-metatarsals IV-V (Lisfranc), Intermetatarsals II-V

1,2. Supination-Pronation of forefoot.

PA (pars anterior)	sitting with leg hanging over edge of table.
Starting position:	Hindfoot and midfoot stabilized.
Plurimeter base:	the Plurimeter is attached to the foot-plate and held firmly against the metatarsal heads. Dial is set at "0⁰" (Neutral-Zero position) supinal pronation. Supination 45⁰, Pronation 15⁰.
Supination:	45⁰
Pronation:	15⁰
SFTR-Recording:	RPA:45-0-15

3. Alternate starting position: prone with knee flexed 90⁰ and foot in anatomical position; the leg, ankle and midfoot are stabilized.

Plurimeter base:	Same as above.
Pronation:	35⁰
SFTR-Recording:	RPA:0-35

4. Extension and flexion of the great toe at the metatarsophalangeal joint (MTP I). S:70-0-45.
5. Metararsus Varus I of 30⁰.   TMT I: F:0-30.
6. Hallux Valgus of 50⁰.
   Position: patient supine, foot in neutral position. Base of Plurimeter parallel to long axis of metatarsal I. Dial is set at 0⁰, then the base is placed over the proximal phalanx and the hallux valgus angle read.
7. Extension and flexion at the metatarsophalangeal joints of second and fifth toes (MTP II-V). Recording: S:40-0-35.
8. Extension and flexion at the proximal interphalangeal joints of second to fifth toes (PIP II-V). Recording: S:0-0-40.
9. Extension and flexion at the distal interphalangeal joints of second to fifth toes (DIP II-V). Recording: S:30-0-55.
   The Plurimeter may be used for forefoot and toe measurements, but it is more convenient to use special custom made goniometers for measurements of the digits.

THE TOES: Abbreviations:

MT	metatarsal bone	MTP	metatarsophalangeal joint
PP	proximal phalanx	PIP	proximal interphalangeal joint
MP	middle phalanx	DIP	distal interphalangeal joint
DP	distal phalanx	IPH	interphalangeal joint of hallux
TMT	tarsometatarsal joint		

Remarks:

     Usually limitation of motion of toes is only estimated and may be expressed in two ways, "the motion of a given toe is 2/3, 1/2, or, 1/3 of normal", or "the motion of a given toe is 1/3, 1/2, or, 2/3 restricted".

94

ARTICULATIONES PEDIS
(PARS ANTERIOR, DIGITI PEDIS)

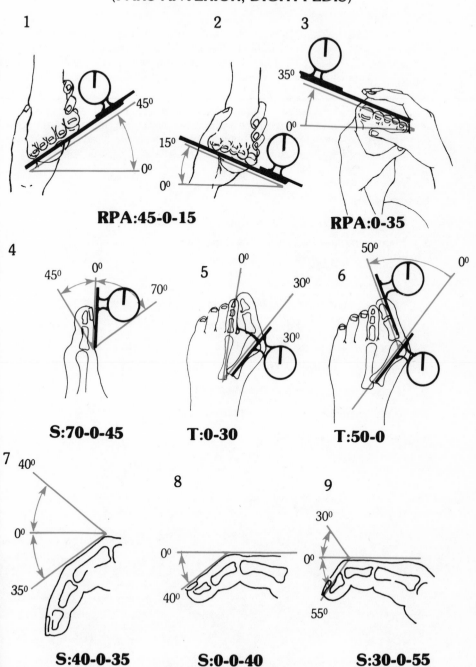

1

45⁰

0⁰

RPA:45-0-15

2

15⁰

0⁰

3

35⁰

0⁰

RPA:0-35

4

45⁰   0⁰   70⁰

S:70-0-45

5

0⁰   30⁰

30⁰

T:0-30

6

50⁰   0⁰

T:50-0

7   40⁰

0⁰

35⁰

S:40-0-35

8

0⁰

40⁰

S:0-0-40

9

30⁰

0⁰

55⁰

S:30-0-55

PLURI-CAL

ADDITIONAL COMPONENTS

The PLURI-CAL (Caliper), is a slide rule with two movable arms -- one horizontal and one vertical. The PLURIMETER can be attached allowing exact positioning of the PLURI-CAL in the horizontal or vertical position. Suitable measurements of diameters and distances, inclinations and tilts can be taken.

The PLURI-CAL allows longitudinal, horizontal and vertical measurements and further measurements of inside and outside diameters, and prosthetic socket dimensions, height differences. The movable arms can be tilted 90°, and there is an attachment for the Pluri-V. An air bubble leveler device is optional.

Examples are:

1. Measurements of pelvic tilt in leg shortening and correcting.
2. Measurement of shortening of the femur.
3. Measurement of the tibia.
4. Measurement of forefoot supination.
5. Measurements of the inside diameter of prosthetic socket.
6. Measurements of the upper thigh diameter and tilt (flexion contracture).
7. Measurement of the tibial torsion.
8. Measurement of shoe lift.
9. Measurement of pelvic inclination of tilt.
10. Measurement of the level of posterior, superior iliac spines.
11. Measurement of rib hump.

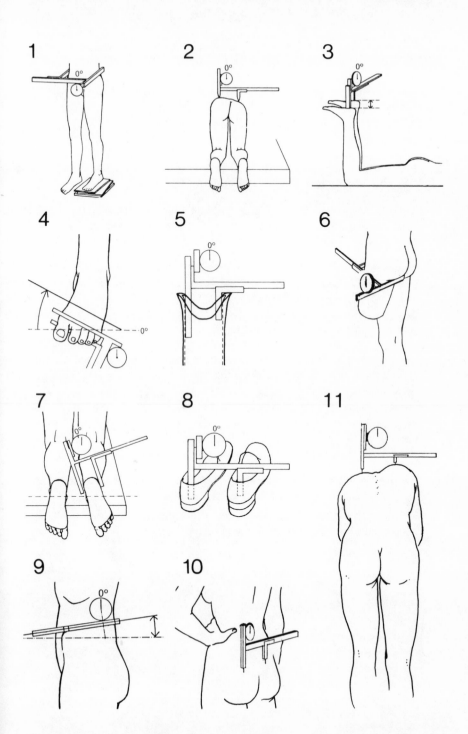

GONIOMETERS AND INCLINOMETERS

BRIEF REVUE OF COMMONLY USED MEASURING INSTRUMENTS.

1. Two-armed goniometer: Wide transparent arms with same width dial. Popular and inexpensive.

   Problem: Small dial, difficult reading of numbers and short arms. It does not allow precise reading.

2. Transparent goniometer: With large dial, is easily readable for clinical use though measuring of finger motion is not possible.

3. Improved goniometer: It has a rotating dial for automatic indication of zero starting position by using a snap-in mechanism, telescopic one arm, and exchangable attachments to other arm for various alignment needs.

4. Single arm inclinometer: Fluid filled without indicator needle (air bubble goniometer). Circular tube is filled with a colored oil and an air bubble indicates constant vertical position.

   Problem: The air bubble is not a precise measuring reference point and readings of degrees are therefore inaccurate.

5. Fluid-level inclinometer: A circular tube is half filled with colored oil. The fluid level indicates a constant horizontal line.

   Problem: There are two reference points but only one can be used, therefore mistakes can occur and measurements are not comparable. Two lines and degrees from 0^0-360^0 makes reading confusing. Starting position other than vertical or horizontal cannot be set. Two instruments and calculations are needed for measuring of the spine.

6. Fluid inclinometer with indicator: The indicator has a small air-filled capsule that constantly points to the vertical position.

   Problem: Relatively large space for the capsule is needed and the fluid filled container becomes bulky and heavy.

1

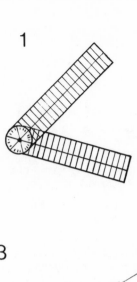

2

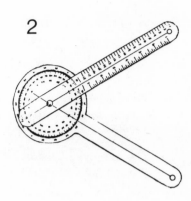

3

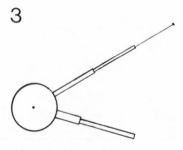

4

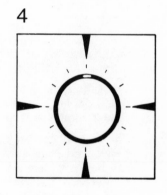

5

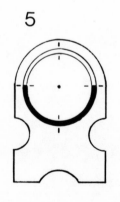

6

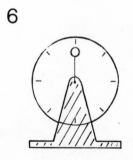

99

FLUID AND ELECTRONIC INCLINOMETERS

1. Fluid inclinometer with counterweighted needle: constantly indicates vertical position.

   Advantages: The counterweight can be very thin and therefore the container is thinner and the instrument is lighter.

   Problem: These are precision instruments and must be cared for properly (exposure to extreme heat, cold or dropping of the instrument must be avoided).

2. The improved version has a rotating dial which snaps in every 90^0; the starting position can be set quickly and precisely.

   The new version also represents a modular system which allows combinations of the instrument with various attachments.

3. Electronic inclinometers: Some are fluid filled which operate like a pendulum inclinometers. The display is easily readable, the zero position can be set quickly. They can be attached to a computer and printer.

   Problem: Expensive, cable connections may be distracting. Electronic digital display does not necessarily secure precision, which depends upon proper components and exact precision mechanics.

4. The state of the art new inclinometer is an electronic digital instrument based upon a capacitive gravity sensor. Active and passive ranges of motion can be easily taken. It has very few controls with no electrodes or cable connections. It is self contained and portable. It has a nine volt battery and can be used up to 100 hrs. Simple attachments for additional measurements are also available.

1

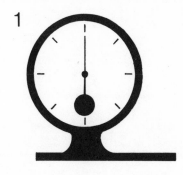

2

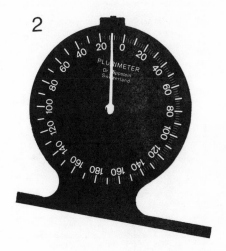

PLURIMETER
Dr. Rippstein
Switzerland

3

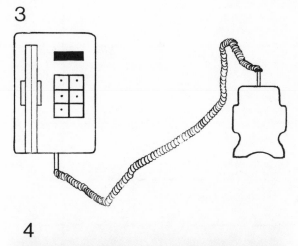

4

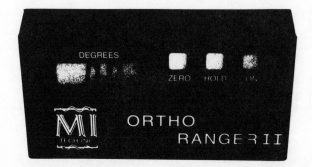

DEGREES

ZERO   HOLD   ON

MI
TECH INC

ORTHO
RANGER II

TABLE OF MOTION

Sym-bol	Group I	Neutral-Zero Starting Position	Group II
S	Extension Hyperextension Dorsiflexion	-0-	Flexion Palmar flexion Plantar flexion
F	Abduction Elevation	-0-	Adduction Depression
F	Radial deviation	-0-	Ulnar deviation
F	Lateral bend to Left of head and trunk (spine)	-0-	Lateral bend to Right of head and trunk (spine)
F	Valgus	-0-	Varus
T	Horizontal extension of shoulder	-0-	Horizontal flexion of shoulder
T	Abduction of hip in 90° flexion	-0-	Adduction of hip in 90° flexion
R	External rotation	-0-	Internal rotation
R	Supination	-0-	Pronation
R	Rotation to Left of head and trunk	-0-	Rotation to Right of head and trunk

TABLE OF MOTION

Sym-bol	Group I	Neutral-Zero Starting Position	Group II
CR (Circum-duction)	Retroposition of metatarsal I (MT I)	-0-	Opposition of metatarsal I (MT I)
VF	Extension of MT I (Radial abduction)	-0-	Flexion of MT I (Radial Adduction)
VS	Abduction of MT I (Palmar abduction)	-0-	Adduction of MT I (Palmar adduction)
FD	Radial deviation of thumb and finger joints	-0-	Ulnar deviation of thumb and finger joints
TD	Abduction of toe joints	-0-	Adduction of toe joints
FC	Valgus of calcaneus	-0-	Varus of calcaneus
F GH	Abduction gleno-humeral joint	-0-	Adduction gleno-humeral joint
F PP	Hindfoot eversion	-0-	Hindfoot inversion
F PM	Midfoot eversion	-0-	Midfoot inversion
R PA	Forefoot supination	-0-	Forefoot pronation
T TM	Pes Metatarsus Valgus (Pes Abductus) Hallux Valgus	-0-	Pes Metatarsus Varus (Pes Adductus) Digitus Quintus Varus

SHOULDER JOINT

Joint	Plane	Motion	Average Range of Motion	Position of Patient	Neutral-Zero Starting Position
S H O U L D E R	S	Extension-0-Flexion glenohumeral and scapular motion	S:50-0-170	Standing or Ext. prone, Flex. supine	Anatomical Arm at side of body
	F	Abduction-0-Adduction	F:170-0-0 (F170-0-75)	Standing, sitting, prone or supine	Anatomical Arm at side of body
	FGH	Abduction-0-Adduction (glenohumeral joint)	FGH 65-0-0	Standing, sitting, prone or supine	Anatomical Arm at side of body
	T	Horizontal-0-Horizontal extension flexion	T:30-0-135	Sitting, prone or supine	Arm extended in 90^0 abduction (F90)
	R (F0)	Ext.Rot.-0-Int.Rot.	R(F0) 60-0-80	Sitting or standing	Arm at side of body with elbow 90^0 flexed
	R (F90)	Ext.Rot.-0-Int.Rot.	R(F90) 90-0-80	Standing, sitting or supine	Humerus 90^0 Abducted, elbow 90^0 flexed

1. Approximate position of the rotational axis of the goniometer indicated in parentheses.

2. Combined gleno-humeral and scapulo-thoracic motion.

3. True adduction blocked by trunk. Adduction beyond 0^0 in front of trunk at about 20^0 flexion.

4. Gleno-humeral motion, only passive: scapula must be stabilized.

5. Horizontal extension is tested in prone, horizontal flexion in supine position.

6. Internal rotation is limited by trunk.

GONIOMETER		Foot-notes	PLURIMETER		Plane
Stationary Arm 1	Movable Arm		Patient's Position	Base	
Parallel to mid-axillary line (humeral head)	Lateral mid-line of humerus	2	Standing, sitting, supine, prone	Over extended fore-arm or arm	S
Parallel to long axis of trunk (variable)	Midline of humerus	3	Standing, sitting, side-lying	On lateral arm	F
Parallel to long axis of trunk (glenohum. joint)	Midline of humerus	4	Standing, sitting, side-lying	On lateral arm, scapula stabilized	FGH
Parallel to shoulder line (acromion)	Parallel to midline of humerus	5	Prone, supine with shoulder over edge of table	Over arm	T
Parallel to fore-arm in starting position	Parallel to long axis of ulna (super-imposed over stat. arm)	6	Side-lying	On lateral forearm	R(F0) Elbow (S90)
Horizontal parallel to forearm in starting position	Parallel to ulna		Standing, sitting or supine	On dorsal or volar forearm	R(F90) Elbow (S90)

SHOULDER GIRDLE-ELBOW-FOREARM-WRIST JOINTS

Joint	Plane	Motion	Average Range of Motion	Position of Patient	Neutral-Zero Starting Position
S G H I O R U D L L D E E R	F	Elevation-0-Depression	F:20-0-10	Sitting or standing	Acromion at level of jugular notch
	T	Retraction-0-Protraction	T:20-0-20	Sitting or standing	Anatomical. Shoulder in F plane
E L B O W	S	Extension-0-Flexion	S:0-0-150	Supine, standing or sitting	Extended arm in anatomical position
	F	Rad.Dev.-0-Uln.Dev. (valgus)　　(varus)	Position Only F:10-0	Supine, standing or sitting	Extended arm in anatomical position
F A O R R M E	R	Supination-0-Pronation	R:90-0-80	Sitting or standing	Arm at side of body elbow 90° flexed, thumb up
W R I S T	S	Extension-0-Flexion	S:50-0-60	Sitting	Wrist extended
	F	Rad.Dev-0-Uln.Dev.	F:20-0-30	Sitting	Wrist extended

1. Primary motion of scapula and clavicle.

2. Overstretching (hyperextension) of e.g. 5° is recorded as: S:5-0-150.

3. Physiological carrying angle of 10° (valgus) equals: F:10-0. Cubitus varus 5° is: F:0-5.

GONIOMETER		Foot-notes	PLURIMETER		Plane
Stationary Arm	Movable Arm		Patient's Position	Base	
Parallel to floor at jugular notch (Rotational axis: jugular notch)	Parallel to jugular notch-acromion line		Sitting or standing	Over acromion, shoulders horizontal	F
Parallel to shoulder line F plane (calvaria)	Calvaria-acromion line	1	Prone, supine with shoulder extended over edge of table	Over ant. shoulder (supine position) or post. shoulder (prone position)	T
Parallel to lateral midline of humerus (elbow)	Parallel to lateral mid-line of radius	2	Standing, sitting, supine	Over lateral fore-arm	S
Parallel to mid-line of humerus (Mid-Cubita)	Parallel to long axis of forearm	3	Sitting, standing, side-lying, arm ab-ducted	Lateral side of arm, or lateral forearm	F
Vertical in F (tip of middle finger)	Parallel to ex-tended thumb	4	Sitting, standing with elbow flexed 90⁰	Across dorsum of wrist. Stabilize wrist in neutral position	R
Parallel to lateral midline of ulna (center of joint)	Parallel to lateral axis of fifth metacarpal	5	Sitting, supine, elbow flexed S90 hand over edge of table	Over dorsum of hand	S
Parallel to mid-line of forearm (center of joint)	Parallel to midline of third metacarpal	6	Supine, or sitting with elbow flexed wrist in neutral position (thumb up)	Parallel to third metacarpal	F

4. Elbow is flexed 90⁰ and close to body; the thumb is in same plane as the distal ulna and radius. Dorsum of hand is parallel to humerus.

5. Elbow should be flexed with no support under arm.

6. Arm 90⁰ abducted, forearm between supination and pronation.

CARPO-METACARPAL JOINT I (CMC I)
METACARPO-PHALANGEAL JOINT I (MCP I)

Joint	Plane	Motion	Average Range of Motion	Position of Patient	Neutral-Zero Starting Position
CMC I	VF	Extension-0-Flexion	VF:20-0-15	Anatomical, fingers extended	Anatomical thumb extended along index finger
	VS	Abduction-0-Adduction	VS:40-0-0	Anatomical, fingers extended	Anatomical thumb extended along index finger
	CR	Retro- -0- Ante-position position MC I MC I	CR:20-0-90	Retroposition: hand prone Anteposition hand supine	Thumb in maximal radial abduction palm stabilized
MCP I	S	Extension-0-Flexion	S(0-10-55)	Hand in neutral rotation	Thumb extended and abducted
	FD	Rad.Dev.-0- Uln.Dev. (abduction adduction) pathological only (ruptured collateral ligaments)	None. Only Pathological	1st metacarpal (MC I) stabilized laterally on table	1st metacarpal (MC I) stabilized laterally on edge of table, thumb extended beyond table
	R	Ext. Rot.-0-Int. Rot.	R:5-0-5	Same as above	Same as above

1. Approximate position of the rotational axis of the goniometer is indicated in parentheses.

2. The extension (or radial abduction), and flexion is recorded as VF (Vector F), the abduction (for palmar abduction), and adduction are recorded as VS (Vector S). Adduction is stopped by metacarpal II.

3. Retroposition and opposition of first metacarpal is measured in two steps.
   Step 1: Retroposition: The hand is stabilized on the table in prone position; the thumb in maximally abducted and lifted up. The angle between table and MC I is measured.
   Step 2: Opposition: The hand is stabilized on the table in supine position; the thumb is maintained in maximal abduction and rotated from the F-plane to the S-plane. The angle between the table and MC I is measured. Retroposition plus Opposition equals Circumduction and is recorded as CR.

4. Pathological radial deviation (abduction) and ulnar deviation (adduction) is found only in laxity or injury (rupture) of collateral ligaments and recorded as FD.

GONIOMETER		Foot-notes	PLURIMETER		Plane
Stationary Arm 1	Movable Arm		Patient's Position	Base	
Parallel to long axis of radius (saddle joint)	Parallel to long axis of metacarpal I	2	Sitting, supine, hand wrist at R0	Over MC I	VF
Parallel to lateral long axis of radius (saddle joint)	Parallel to long axis of metacarpal I	2	Sitting, hand supine	On MC I	VS
Parallel to long axis of first metacarpal (MC I) Exact measure-	Parallel to long axis of MC I	3	Retroposition: Sitting with hand prone , stabilized on table Anteposition same with hand supine	Over extended long axis of MC I	CR
Parallel to long axis of first metacarpal (MC I) (variable)	Parallel to long axis of proximal phalanx (PP)		Sitting with hand in S plane	Over proximal phalanx of thumb	S
Over long axis of MC I	Over long axis of proximal phalanx of thumb	4	MC I in lateral position (45⁰ in relation to palm) stabilized on edge of table, thumb extended beyond table	Lateral base over long axis of proximal phalanx of thumb	FD
Cannot be measured (Plurimeter only)			Same as above	Stabilized across proximal phalanx of thumb	R

INTERPHALANGEAL JOINT OF THE THUMB (POLLEX) IPP

Joint	Plane	Motion	Average Range of Motion	Position of Patient	Neutral-Zero Starting Position
IPP THUMB	S	Extension-0-Flexion	S:15-0-80	Anatomical	Anatomical
	FD	Rad. Dev.-0-Uln. Dev.	S:0-0-0	1st metacarpal (MC I) stabilized laterally on table	1st metacarpal (MC I) stabilized laterally on edge of table, thumb extended beyond table
	R	Ext. Rot.-0-Int. Rot.	R:5-0-5	Same as above	Same as above

4. Pathological radial deviation (abduction) and ulnar deviation (adduction) is found only in laxity or injury (rupture) of collateral ligaments and recorded as FD.

5. IPP equals interphalangeal joint of the thumb (pollex).

GONIOMETER		Foot-notes	PLURIMETER		Plane
Stationary Arm	Movable Arm		Patient's Position	Base	
Over long axis of MC I	Over long axis of distal phalanx	4	Sitting with hand in S plane Proximal phalanx of thumb stabi-lized on table distal beyond table	Over distal phalanx	S
Parallel to long axis of proximal phalanx of thumb	Parallel to long axis of distal phalanx (DP)	5	Same as above, but proximal of thumb is stabi-lized in later-al position.	Lateral over long axis of distal phalanx of thumb	FD
Cannot be measured (Plurimeter only)		4	Same as above	Stabilized across distal phalanx of thumb	R

METACARPO-PHALANGEAL JOINTS II-V (MCP II-V)
PROXIMAL-INTERPHALANGEAL JOINTS II-V (PIP II-V)

Joint	Plane	Motion	Average Range of Motion	Position of Patient	Neutral-Zero Starting Position
MCP II-V	S	Extension-0-Flexion	45-0-90	Anatomical	Anatomical
	F (FD)	Abduction-0-Adduction	Average 30-0-25 variable	Hand pronated, finger closed	Middle finger fixed in extension line of long axis of MC III
	R	Ext.Rot-0-Int.Rot.	5-0-5	Hand in pronation	Anatomical
PIP II-V	S	Extension-0-Flexion	5-0-100	Anatomical	Anatomical
	FD	Abduction-0-Adduction	0-0-0	Hand pronated	Hand pronated
	R	Ext.Rot.-0-Int.Rot Pathological only	5-0-5	Hand pronated	Anatomical

1. Approximate position of the rotational axis of the goniometer is indicated in parentheses.

2. Routine abduction and adduction measurements as related to middle finger (record F). If absolute measurements are taken, refer to radial and ulnar deviation and record "FD" (dorsiflex adjacent fingers to make room for motion).

GONIOMETER		Foot-notes	PLURIMETER		Plane
Stationary Arm 1	Moveable arm		Patient's Position	Base	
Parallel to long axis of metacarpal II-V	Parallel to long axis of proximal phalanx II-V	3	Sitting with hand stabilized on table, fingers extended beyond table	Over proximal phalanx II-V	S
Parallel to long axis of metacarpal III (variable)	Parallel to long axis of finger	2 3	Sitting with hand stabilized in S plane	Lateral over proximal phalanx II-V. Metacarpals stabilized	F (FD)
Cannot be measured (Plurimeter only)			Sitting with hand stabilized on table fingers extended beyond table	Across distal end of proxi-mal phalanx II-V	R
Parallel to long axis of prox-imal phalanx. (center of PIP)	Parallel to long axis of middle phalanx	3	Sitting with hand stabilized on table fingers extended beyond table	Over middle phalanx, prox. phalanx II-V stabilized	S
Same as above	Same as above		Sitting with hand in S-plane	Lateral over middle phalanx, prox. phalanx stabilized	FD
Cannot be measured (Plurimeter only)			Sitting with hand stabilized on table fingers extended beyond table	Across distal end of middle phal. II-V, prox. phal. stabilized	R

3. S and F can be measured more easily with the PLURI-DIG (Plurimeter-Digital).

DISTAL-INTERPHALANGEAL JOINTS II-V (DIP II-V)

Joint	Plane	Motion	Average Range of Motion	Position of Patient	Neutral-Zero Starting Position
DIP II-V	S	Extension-0-Flexion	0-0-60	Anatomical	Anatomical
	FD	Abduction-0-Adduction Pathological only	0-0-0	Hand pronated	Hand pronated
	R	Ext.Rot.-0-Int.Rot.	3-0-3	Hand pronated	Anatomical

GONIOMETER		Foot-Notes	PLURIMETER		Plane
Stationary Arm	Moveable arm		Patient' Position	Base	
Parallel to long axis middle phalanx (center of DIP)	Parallel to long axis of distal phalanx		Sitting with hand stabilized on table. II-V fingers extended beyond table	Over distal phalanx II-V	S
On middle phalanx	On distal phalanx		Sitting with hand in S-plane	Lateral over distal phalanx II-V. Middle phal. stab.	FD
Cannot be measured (Plurimeter only)			Sitting with hand stabilized on table. II-V fingers extended beyond table	Across distal phalanx II-V	R

JOINTS OF THE
CERVICAL SPINE-THORACIC SPINE (CS, TS)

Joint	Plane	Motion	Average Range of Motion	Position of Patient	Neutral-Zero Starting Position
C E R V I C A L S P I N E	S	Exten. -0- Flex.	S:40-0-40	Sitting or standing	Anatomical Position
	F	Lat. -0- Lat. Bend Bend to to Left Right	F:45-0-45	Sitting or standing	Anatomical Position
	R	Rot. -0- Rot. to to Left Right	R:30-0-85	Sitting or standing	Anatomical Position
T H O R A C I C S P I N E	S	Exten. -0- Flex.	S:30-0-85	Extension: Standing or prone Flexion: Standing or supine	Anatomical Position
	F	Lat. -0- Lat. Bend Bend to to Left Right	F:30-0-30	Standing	Anatomical Position
	R	Rot. -0- Rot. to to Left Right	R:45-0-45	Sitting Spine: trunk supported beyond table, pelvis stabilized	Anatomical Position

True Lumbar Spine equals Total lumbar spine motion minus hip motion.

1. Approximate position of the rotational axis of the goniometer is indicated in parentheses.

2. Accurate measuring is very difficult. X-ray, special scoliometer of Debrunner's, inclinometer, pendulum, bubble type instruments, or functional measurement may be used. S-plane: distance in cm chin to jugular notch. F-plane: distance in cm earlobe to acromion.

GONIOMETER		Foot-notes	PLURIMETER		P l a n e
Stationary Arm 1	Movable Arm		Patient's Position	Base	
Parallel to long axis of trunk (variable)	Parallel to long axis of head	2	Standing, sitting	Stabilized on calvaria in S plane	S
Parallel to long axis of trunk (C7 spin.)	Parallel to C7 calvaria line		Standing, sitting	Stabilized on calvaria in F plane	F
Right angle to shoulder line (calvaria)	Parallel to occipito-nasal line		Supine	Stabilized on forehead (in T plane)	R
Parallel to long axis of trunk (about 3 finger breadths below iliac crests)	Parallel to mid-axillary line through spinous process C7	3	Flexion: Standing Extension: Standing or prone (sphinx) position	Stabilized on T1 between scapulae in S plane	S
Parallel to long axis of trunk (L5-S1)	L5-C7 line	3	Standing	Stabilized between scapulae on T1 parallel to floor in F plane	F
Cannot be measured (Plurimeter only)		3	A: Standing with trunk bent. B: Supine, trunk beyond table pelvis stabilized by belt or assistant	A: Stabilized on T1 B: Stabilized on sternum in T plane	R

3. Accurate clinical measurements are not possible. X-ray, special instruments such as scoliometer of Debrunner or functional measurements are more reliable. Flexion and lateral bending: distance in cm finger-tips to floor. Stabilize pelvis and take into consideration different ranges of motion at different levels of the spine. Rotation is almost entirely in the thoracic and minimal in the lumbar spine.

JOINTS OF THE LUMBAR SPINE (LS)

Joint	Plane	Motion	Average Range of Motion	Position of Patient	Neutral Zero Starting Position
L U M B A R S P I N E	S	Extension-0-Flexion	S:30-0-45	Standing	Anatomical
	F	Lat. -0- Lat. bend bend to to left right	F:25-0-25	Standing	Anatomical
	R	Ext. Rot.-0- Int. Rot.	R:5-0-5	Standing trunk bent over	Anatomical

3. Accurate clinical measurements are not possible. X-ray, special instruments such as scoliometer of Debrunner or functional measurements are more reliable. Flexion and lateral bending: distance in cm fingertips to floor. Stabilize pelvis and take into consideration different ranges of motion at different levels of the spine. Rotation is almost entirely in the thoracic and minimal in the lumbar spine.

| GONIOMETER | | Foot-notes | PLURIMETER | | Plane |
Stationary Arm	Movable Arm		Patient's Position	Base	
No accurate measurements can be taken with conventional goniometer (Plurimeter only)		3	Standing	First on L1 then on sacrum	S
		3	Standing	Stabilized over L1	F
		3	Standing trunk bent forword	On upper LS across L1	R

HIP JOINT

Joint	Plane	Motion	Average Range of Motion	Position of Patient	Neutral-Zero Starting Position
H I P	S	Extension-0-Flexion	S:15-0-125	Extension: prone Flexion: supine	Hip in anatomical position, knee flexed
	S	Straight Leg Raising (SLR)-, Lasseque test Neutral-Zero to flexion	Neutral-Zero to pain threshold	Supine knee extended or sitting (knee flexed)	Hip and knee extended Hip and knee flexed 90°
	F	Abduction-0-Adduction 1	F:45-0-35	Supine	Extended leg anatomical position
	T	Abduction-0-Adduction in 90° hip in 90° hip flexion flexion	T:45-0-20	Supine standing or sitting	Thigh in 90° flexion between abduction and adduction
	R	Ext. Rot. -0- Int. Rot. (standard position) Hip S90 Knee S90	R:45-0-35	Sitting hip and knee flexed 90° over edge of table	Midway between external-internal rotation
	R	Ext. Rot. -0- Int. Rot. Hip S0 Knee S90	R:45-0-40	1. Supine 2. Prone hip extended knee flexed 90° over edge of table	Midway between external-internal rotation
	R	Ext. Rot. -0- Int. Rot. Hip S0 Knee S0	R:45-0-40	Supine; Hip and knee extended	Midway between external-internal rotation

1. Abduction of the leg should be measured by the Pluri-Tel

120

GONIOMETER		Foot-notes	PLURIMETER		Plane
Stationary Arm	Movable Arm		Patient's Position	Base	
Line greater trochanter-iliac crest parallel to trunk. Rotational axis greater trochanter	Lateral midline of femur		Supine with opposite hip flexed	On thigh in S plane	S
Parallel to table and lateral axis of femur	over long axis of thigh (knee extended)		supine with knee extended (SLR, Lasseque)	On thigh in S plane On tibia in S plane	S Knee (S0)
Parallel to connecting left and right anterior superior iliac spine	Mechanical axis of the thigh	1	Side-lying upper thigh parallel to table	On lateral thigh just above knee or over longitudinal axis of thigh when using PLURI-TEL	F
Anterior-posterior horizontal line plane (tub. oss. ischii).	Midline of thigh		Standing, side-lying, supine Hip flexed in S plane	Stabilized on knee parallel to table, knee and hip flexed 90°	T
1. Parallel to long axis of trunk or 2. perpendicular to floor (knee)	Midline of tibia (leg)		Sitting	On leg or parallel to axis of tibia	F S90 Knee S90
Perpendicular to floor (knee)	Midline of tibia		Prone	On leg as above	R S90 Knee S90
Perpendicular to floor (tuber calcanei)	Long axis of foot		Supine	Lateral on long axis of foot with ankle and knee stabilized	R (S0) Knee

KNEE-LEG-ANKLE JOINTS

Joint	Plane	Motion	Average Range of Motion	Position of Patient	Neutral-Zero Starting Position
K N E E	S	Extension-0-Flexion	S:0-0-130	Sitting	Extended knee anatomical
	F	Valgus-0-Varus	Position only	Supine or standing (weight-bearing)	Extended knee anatomical
L E G	R	Ext. Rot.-0- Int. Rot.	R:20-0-10	Sitting leg hanging free	Knee S90 Ankle S0
A N K L E	S	Extension-0-Flexion (Dorsi-flexion) (Plantar-flexion)	S:20-0-45	Sitting, supine or prone	Anatomical Hip S0 or S90 Knee S90

1. Approximate position of the rotational axis of the goniometer is indicated in parentheses.

2. Axis varies in different positions.

3. For Neutral-Zero Starting Position, use mechanical axis of thigh line connecting middle of femoral head with center of knee extended. Physiological varus of infant and valgus of adult.

4. Leg hanging free, foot at 90° in relation to tibia midway between external and internal rotation and eversion and inversion (stabilize latter at lower ankle joint). Motion occurs at knee and ankle joints.

5. Keep arms of goniometer well aligned - axis will change. Keep foot midway between eversion and inversion. Motion in upper ankle joint (talocrural).

GONIOMETER		Foot-notes	PLURIMETER		Plane
Stationary Arm 1	Movable Arm		Patient's Position	Base	
Parallel to lateral midline of femur	Parallel to lateral midline of fibula	2	Sitting	On distal tibia or heel	S
Mechanical axis of hip and thigh center of joint	Long axis of tibia	3	Standing	Over long axis of femur-set to 0-, then over long axis of tibia	F
Anteroposterior horizontal line (tuber calcanei)	Parallel to long axis of foot	4	Prone, supine	On heel, ankle stabilized	R
Parallel to lateral midline of fibula (variable)	Lateral midline of fifth metatarsal	5	Sitting, supine	On plantar side of heel	S

HEEL-HINDFOOT-MIDFOOT-FOREFOOT JOINTS

Joint	Plane	Motion	Average Range of Motion	Position of Patient	Neutral-Zero Starting Position
HEEL	FC	Valgus -0- Varus	5-0-5	Standing	Long axis of leg (tibia) heel vertical
HIND FOOT	FPP	Eversion -0- Inversion Hindfoot	10-0-20	Supine, sitting	Anatomical
MID FOOT	FPM	Eversion-0-Inversion Midfoot	5-0-5	Supine, sitting	Anatomical
FORE FOOT	RPA	Supination -0- Pronation Forefoot	30-0-20	Sitting, standing	Anatomical
	S	Extension -0- Flexion	Usually position only	Anatomical	Anatomical
	T	Abduction -0- Adduction (Valgus -0- Varus)	Same as above	Anatomical	Anatomical

1. Approximate position of the rotational axis of the goniometer is indicated in parentheses.

2. Leg should be stabilized or knee flexed to avoid hip rotation. Motion in lower ankle joint (subtalar), and transverse tarsal and midtarsal joints.

3. As above, but motion in midtarsal joints only.

4. Passive motion in subtalar joint only, or position to record degree of eversion (valgus, pronation), or inversion (varus, supination), of heel with weight bearing.

5. Metatarsale varum I: angle between long axis of MT I and MT II.

GONIOMETER		Foot-notes	PLURIMETER		Plane
Stationary Arm 1	Movable Arm		Patient's Position	Base	
Parallel to long axis of leg (tibia)	Parallel to vertical axis of heel	4	Standing, sitting	Parallel to vertical calcaneal axis or use caliper, stabilize tibia	F
Parallel to long axis of tibia	Parallel to vertical cal-caneal axis	2	Sitting or prone with knee flexed and stabilized	Stabilized on heel (plantar) or used on caliper. Ankle stabilized	FPP
Cannot be measured (Plurimeter only)			Same as above	Stabilized on midfoot (plantar) or used on caliper. Hindfoot stabilized.	FPM
Parallel to long axis of tibia	Across meta-tarsals	3	Same as above	On sole across MT heads or caliper. Hindfoot and mid-foot stabilized	RPA
Parallel to long axis of hindfoot and midfoot	Parallel to metatarsals		Same as above	First on plantar side of hind and midfoot, position on 0⁰, then on metatarsals	S
Same as above in T plane	Parallel to metatarsals	5	Supine, prone or side-lying	Parallel to long axis of hind and midfoot. Set dial on 0⁰ and apply base parallel to metatarsals	T

METATARSO-PHALANGEAL JOINT I (MTP I)
INTERPHALANGEAL I (IPH) JOINT OF THE BIG TOE
(HALLUX)

Joint	Plane	Motion	Average Range of Motion	Position of Patient	Neutral-Zero Starting Position
MTP I	S	Extension-0-Flexion	60-0-40	Sitting or supine. Big toe in anatomical position	Anatomical
	T	Abduction-0-Adduction	20-0-20	Sitting or supine. Big toe in anatomical position	Anatomical
	R	Ext. Rot.-0- Int. Rot.	3-0-3	Sitting or supine. Big toe in anatomical position	Anatomical
IPH	S	Extension-0-Flexion	0-0-60	Sitting or supine	Anatomical
	T	Abduction-0-Adduction	0-0-0	Sitting or supine	Anatomical
	R	Ext. Rot.-0- Int. Rot.	3-0-3	Sitting or supine	Anatomical

Joints of the Hindfoot: talo-calcaneal and talo-calcaneo-navicular joints.

Joints of the Midfoot: talo-calcaneo-navicular, calcaneo-cuboid, cuneo-cuboid, intercuneiform, cuneo-navicular joints.

Joints of the Forefoot: cuneo-metatarsal II-III, intermetatarsal II-III and III-V, cuneiform I-metatarsal I, cuboid-metatarsal IV-V joints.

1. Hallux Valgus: angle between long axis of MT I and proximal phalanx of great toe (abduction in MTP joint).

2. Digitus Quintus Varus: angle between long axis of MT V and proximal phalanx of little toe (adduction in MTP joint).

GONIOMETER		Foot- notes	PLURIMETER		Plane
Stationary Arm	Movable Arm		Patient's Position	Base	
Over meta-tarsal I	Over proxi-mal phalanx	1, 2	Sitting or supine. Foot and big toe in anatomi-cal position	Over proxi-mal phalanx	S
Over meta-tarsal I	Over proxi-mal phalanx		Sitting or supine. Foot and big toe in anatomi-cal position	Over proxi-mal phalanx	T
Cannot be measured (Plurimeter only)			Sitting or supine. Foot and big toe in anatomi-cal position	Across proximal phalanx	R
Over proxi-mal phalanx	Over distal phalanx		Sitting or supine	Over distal phalanx	S
Over proxi-mal phalanx	Over distal phalanx		Sitting or supine	Over distal phalanx	T
Cannot be measured (Plurimeter only)			Sitting or supine	Across dis-tal phalanx	R

METATARSO-PHALANGEAL JOINTS II-V (MTP II-V)
PROXIMAL INTERPHALANGEAL JOINTS II-V (PIP II-V)

Joint	Plane	Motion	Average Range of Motion	Position of Patient	Neutral Zero Starting Position
MTP II-V	S	Extension-0-Flexion	60-0-40	Sitting or supine. Foot and toes in anatomical position	Anatomical
	T	Abduction-0-Adduction	30-0-20	Sitting or supine. Foot and toes in anatomical position	Anatomical
	R	Ext. Rot.-0- Int. Rot.	3-0-3	Sitting or supine. Foot and toes in anatomical position	Anatomical
PIP II-V	S	Extension-0-Flexion	5-0-40	Sitting or supine	Anatomical
	T	Abduction-0-Adduction	0-0-0	Sitting or supine	Anatomical
	R	Ext. Rot.-0- Int. Rot.	3-0-3	Sitting or supine	Anatomical

Joints of the Hindfoot: talo-calcaneal and talo-calcaneo-navicular joints.

Joints of the Midfoot: talo-calcaneo-navicular, calcaneo-cuboid, cuneo-cuboid, intercuneiform, cuneo-navicular joints.

Joints of the Forefoot: cuneo-metatarsal II-III, intermetatarsal II-III and III-V, cuneiform I-metatarsal I, cuboid-metatarsal IV-V joints.

1. Hallux Valgus: angle between long axis of MT I and proximal phalanx of great toe (abduction in MTP joint).

2. Digitus Quintus Varus: angle between long axis of MT V and proximal phalanx of little toe (adduction in MTP joint).

128

GONIOMETER		Foot-notes	PLURIMETER		Plane
Stationary Arm	Movable Arm		Patient's Position	Base	
Over metatarsal II-V	Over proximal phalanx	1, 2	Sitting or supine. Foot and toes in anatomical position	Over proximal phalanx	S
Over metatarsal II-V	Over proximal phalanx		Sitting or supine. Foot and toes in anatomical position	Over proximal phalanx	T
Cannot be measured (Plurimeter only)			Sitting or supine. Foot and toes in anatomical position	Across proximal phalanx	R
Over proximal phalanx	Over medial phalanx		Sitting or supine. Foot in anatomical position	Over medial phalanx	S
Over proximal phalanx	Over medial phalanx		Sitting or supine	Over medial phalanx	T
Cannot be measured (Plurimeter only)			Sitting or supine	Across medial phalanx	R

DISTAL-INTERPHALANGEAL JOINTS II-V (DIP II-V)

Joint	Plane	Motion	Average Range of Motion	Position of Patient	Neutral Zero Starting Position
DIP II-V	S	Extension-0-Flexion	0-0-50	Sitting or supine	Anatomical
	T	Abduction-0-Adduction	0-0-0	Sitting or supine	Anatomical
	R	Ext. Rot.-0- Int. Rot.	3-0-3	Sitting or supine	Anatomical

Joints of the Hindfoot: talo-calcaneal and talo-calcaneo-navicular joints.

Joints of the Midfoot: talo-calcaneo-navicular, calcaneo-cuboid, cuneo-cuboid, intercuneiform, cuneo-navicular joints.

Joints of the Forefoot: cuneo-metatarsal II-III, intermetatarsal II-III and III-V, cuneiform I-metatarsal I, cuboid-metatarsal IV-V joints.

1. Hallux Valgus: angle between long axis of MT I and proximal phalanx of great toe (abduction in MTP joint).
2. Digitus Quintus Varus: angle between long axis of MT V and proximal phalanx of little toe (adduction in MTP joint).

GONIOMETER		Foot-notes	PLURIMETER		Plane
Stationary Arm	Movable Arm		Patient's Position	Base	
Over medial phalanx	Over distal phalanx	1, 2	Sitting or supine. Foot in anatomical position	Over proximal phalanx	S
Over medial phalanx	Over distal phalanx		Sitting or supine	Over distal phalanx	T
Cannot be measured (Plurimeter only)			Sitting or supine	Across distal phalanx	R

MOST IMPORTANT MEASUREMENTS
OF THE UPPER EXTREMITY

Joint	Plane	Right	Left
Shoulder			
Extension/Flexion	S	55-0-170	55-0-170
Abduction/Adduction	F	175-0-50	175-0-50
Horizontal Extension/Horizontal Flexion			
Arm in 90° Abduction	T	30-0-135	30-0-135
External Rotation/Internal Rotation			
Arm at side	R(F0)	60-0-70	60-0-70
Arm in 90° Abduction	R(F90)	90-0-80	90-0-80
Elbow			
Extension/Flexion	S	0-0-145	0-0-145
Forearm Rotation			
Supination/Pronation	R	90-0-80	90-0-80
Wrist			
Extension/Flexion	S	70-0-80	70-0-80
Radial Deviation/Ulnar Deviation	F	20-0-40	20-0-40

Fingers

Usually functional measurements (fingertip-distal crease of the palm distance, etc).

Circumferential Measurements:

In comparison with the good side, circumferences are measured at the elbow, 15 cm above and below proximal and distal, the ulnar epicondyle of the humerus, also at the wrist level and the metacarpals (MC II-V). For measurements on amputees and for fitting of compression sleeves, measurements are taken in one inch increments.

Linear Measurements:

In amputees, the length of the stump as well as the good arm is recorded. Reference points are bony prominences that are palpable under the skin such as the acromion, medial epicondyle of the humerus, tip of the olecranon, styloid process of radius, metacarpo-phalangeal joint and tip of the fingers; in presence of fingerstumps, tracing of the hand with fingers abducted is used.

MOST IMPORTANT MEASUREMENTS
OF THE LOWER EXTREMITY

Joint	Plane	Right	Left
Hip			
Extension/Flexion	S	25-0-125	25-0-125
Abduction/Adduction	F	50-0-30	50-0-30
Ext. Rotation/Int. Rotation			
Hip extended	R(S0)	45-0-40	45-0-40
Hip 90° flexed	R(S90)	45-0-40	45-0-40
Knee			
Extension/Flexion	S	0-0-135	0-0-135
Ankle (upper ankle joint)			
Extension/Flexion (plantar)	S	20-0-50	20-0-50
Heel (Calcaneus)			
Valgus-0-Varus	FC	5-0-5	5-0-5
Hindfoot			
Eversion/Inversion	FPP	10-0-20	10-0-20
Midfoot			
Eversion/Inversion	FPM	5-0-5	5-0-5
Forefoot			
Supination/Pronation	RPA	30-0-20	30-0-20

Circumferential Measurements:
The measurements taken most frequently are 10 cm and 20 cm above and 15 cm below the medial joint space of the knee, over the proximal border of the patella, over the knee joint proper, over the maximum circumference of the calf, minimal circumference above the ankle and over the malleoli. Comparison with the other side is always made. For stump measurements (shrinking) measurements are taken in one inch increments.

Longitudinal Measurements:
In amputees, length measurements of the stump as well as of the remaining extremity are made. Reference points again are bony prominences that are palpable under the skin: anterior superior iliac spine, ischial tuberosity, major trochantor, medial or lateral joint space of the knee, tip of the medial or lateral malleolus, heel, tip of the big toe. Measurements of relative length of the lower extremity: umbilicus - tip of medial malleolus.

AVERAGE RANGES OF MOTION

Cervical Spine
   Extension/Flexion
   Lateral Bending to the Left/Right
   Rotation to the Left/Right

S	40-0-40
F	45-0-45
R	50-0-50

Thoracic and Lumbar Spine
   Extension/Flexion
   Lateral Bending to the Left/Right
   Rotation to the Left/Right

S	30-0-85
F	30-0-30
R	45-0-45

Shoulder
   Extension/Flexion
   Abduction/Adduction
   Horizontal Extension/Horizontal Flexion
   Ext. Rotation/Int. Rotation
      Arm at side
      Arm in 90° Abduction

S	50-0-170
F	170-0-75
T	30-0-135
R(F0)	60-0-70
R(F90)	90-0-80

Elbow
   Extension/Flexion

S	0-0-150

Forearm
   Supination/Pronation

R	90-0-80

Wrist
   Extension/Flexion
   Radial Deviation/Ulnar Deviation

S	50-0-60
F	20-0-30

Hip
   Extension/Flexion
   Abduction/Adduction (Hip extended)
   Abduction/Adduction (Hip in 90° Flexion)
   Ext. Rotation/Int. Rotation
      Hip and Knee extended
      Hip and Knee in 90° Flexion

S	15-0-125
F	45-0-15
T	45-0-20
R(S0)	45-0-40
R(S90)	45-0-45

Knee
   Extension/Flexion
   Abduction, valgus/Adduction, varus

S	0-0-130
F	0-0-0

Ankle Joint		
Extension/Flexion	S	20-0-50
Abduction/Adduction (heel valgus/varus)	FC	5-0-5

Foot		
Hindfoot Eversion/Inversion	FPP	10-0-20
Midfoot Eversion/Inversion	FPM	5-0-5
Forefoot Supination/Pronation	RPA	30-0-20

Big Toe		
MTP I Extension/Flexion	S	60-0-40
Abduction/Adduction (hallux valgus)	T	20-0-20
Ext. Rot./Int. Rot.	R	3-0-3

IPH		
Extension/Flexion	S	0-0-60
Abduction/Adduction	T	0-0-0
Ext. Rot./Int. Rot.	R	3-0-3

Toes
MTP II-V		
Extension/Flexion	S	60-0-40
Abduction/Adduction (digitus V varus)	T	30-0-20
Ext. Rot./Int. Rot.	R	3-0-3

PIP II-V		
Extension/Flexion	S	5-0-40
Abduction/Adduction	T	0-0-0
Ext. Rot./Int. Rot.	R	3-0-3

DIP II-V		
Extension/Flexion	S	0-0-50
Abduction/Adduction	T	0-0-0
Ext. Rot./Int. Rot.	R	3-0-3

RECORDING OF STRENGTH OF MUSCLE GROUPS IN THE SFTR-METHOD

The SFTR-Method allows brief recording of strength of agonists and antagonists by using standardized numbers 0-5 for expression of strength.

Table of numbers indicating muscle strength according to international standard:

Numbers:		Description	Impairment (%)
5	Normal	Complete Range of Motion (ROM) against gravity and full resistance	0%
4	Good	Complete ROM against gravity and some resistance or reduced force movements and motor control	5-20%
3	Fair	Complete ROM against gravity and only without resistance	25-50%
2	Poor	Complete ROM with gravity eliminated	55-75%
1	Trace	Slight contractibility but no joint motion	80-90%
0	Zero	No contractibility	100%

The hyphens between the anatomical starting position and the two ranges of motion are substituted with directional vectors:

S: EXTENSION-0-FLEXION (Extensors / Flexors)   F: ABDUCTION-0-ADDUCTION (Abductors / Adductors)

R: EXT. ROTATION-0-INT. ROTATION (External rotators / Internal rotators)

The numbers indicating strength are placed above and below the vectors according to the direction of functional motion. If a rule is adopted that agonists (motion recorded to the left of 0), are recorded above the hyphens and antagonists (motions recorded to the right of 0), are recorded below the hyphens, no arrows would be necessary. For example, full strength of extensors and flexors of the shoulder with free range of motion would be recorded as:

$$S:50\frac{5}{5}0\frac{5}{5}180 \qquad S:50-\frac{5}{5}-0-\frac{5}{5}-180$$

To facilitate computer data input, a slash can be used to seperate the numbers expressing strength. The number representing the agonist would precede the slash: the antagonist would follow the slash. This will eliminate the use of superscript and subscript numbers. In the above example, the recording would be:

S:50-5/5-0-5/5-180

136

EXAMPLE OF RECORDING OF RANGE OF MOTION AND STRENGTH OF THE RIGHT SHOULDER

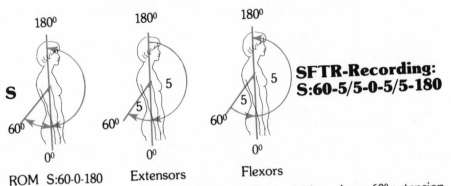

S

ROM S:60-0-180   Extensors   Flexors

SFTR-Recording: S:60-5/5-0-5/5-180

The range of motion of the right shoulder in the S-Plane shows 60° extension and 180° flexion. The extensors and flexors have full strengths (5/5).

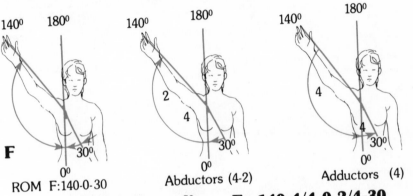

F

ROM F:140-0-30   Abductors (4-2)   Adductors (4)

SFTR-Recording: Fa:140-4/4-0-2/4-30

The active range of motion of the right shoulder in the F-Plane shows restriction of abduction to 140°. The abductors are good in the initial abduction (4), but becoming poor at the terminal range (2). The adductors are good (4). Fa(F-Plane, active).

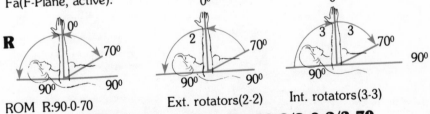

R

ROM R:90-0-70   Ext. rotators(2-2)   Int. rotators(3-3)

SFTR-Recording: Rp:90-2/3-0-2/3-70

The passive external rotation of the right shoulder is 90°, the internal rotation is possible to 70°. The strengths of the external rotators is poor (2) and of the internal rotators fair (3).

Rp(Rotation, passive): active external rotation (against gravity), is not possible because of weak external rotators.

Bibliography

1. American Academy of Orthopaedic Surgeons: Joint Motion Method of Measuring and Recording, Chicago, 1965.

2. American Medical Association: A Guide to the Evaluation of Permanent Impairment of the Extremities and Back, J.A.M.A., Special Edition, Feburary 15, 1958, GUIDES TO THE EVALUATION OF PERMANENT IMPAIRMENT, 1971, 1988.

3. A.U.V.A. Allgemeine Unfallversicherungsanstalt: Neutral-0-Methode, SFTR Notierung, Wien, 1972.

4. Cave, E.F., Roberts, S.M.: A Method of Measuring and Recording Joint Function, Jnl. of Bone and Joint Surg. 18:2, 455-466 April, 1936.

5. Cobb, J.H.: Outline for the Study of Scoliosis. In: Instructional Course Lectures. Amer. Acad. Orthop. Surg., 5-261, 1948.

6. Debrunner, H.U.: Gelenkmessung, Längenmessung, Umfangmessung (Neutral -0-Methode), Bulletin, Offizielles Organ der Schweizersichen Arbeitsgemeinschaft für Osteosynthesefragen, April, 1971.

7. Debrunner, H.U.: Messmethoden in der Orthopaedie unter Berücksichtigung der Internationalen Vorschläge, Verh. Dtsch. Orthop. Ges., 54. Kongr.: 341-350, 1968.

8. Debrunner, H.U., Müller, M.E.: Orthopaediches Diagnostikum, Bilder, Übersichten, Tabellen, Georg Thieme, Verlag, Stuttgart, 1966, 1973, 1976.

9. Gerhardt, J.J.: International Standard Orthopedic Measurements Wall Chart, Orthopedic Equipment Company, Bourbon, Indiana, U.S.A., 1964.

10. Gerhardt, J.J.: Clinical Measurements of Joint Motion and Position in the Neutral-Zero Method and SFTR Recording: Basic Principles. Journal International Rehabilitation Medicine Association, Eular Publishers, Basel, Switzerland, 1983.

11. Gerhardt, J.J., King, P.S., Zettl, J.H.: Immediate and Early Prosthetic Management, Rehabilitation Aspects, pp. 239-275. Hans Huber Publishers, Toronto, Lewiston, N.Y., Bern, Stuttgart, 1986.

12. Gerhardt, J.J., Reiner, E., Schwaiger, B., King, P.S.: Interdisciplinary Rehabilitation in Trauma. pp. 571-597. Williams and Wilkins, Baltimore, London, Los Angeles, Sydney, 1987.

13. Hellebrandt, F.A., Duvall, E.N., Moore, M.L.: The Measurements of Joint Motion, Part III-Reliability of Goniometry, Phys. Ther. Rev. 29:302-307. July, 1949.

14. Kapandji, I.A.: The Physiology of Joints, Vol. I, Upper Limb, Lower Limb, Churchill Livingston, Edinburgh, London, New York, 1970.

15. Kapandji, I.A.: The Physiology of the Joints, Vol 3, The Trunk and The Vertebral Column, Churchill Livingston, Edinburgh, London, New York, 1974.

16. Kiszel, S.: Die Lateinische Diagnose in der Unfallchirurgie und ihren Grenzgebieten (Diagnosenverzeichnis), Allgemeine Unfallversicherungsanstalt, A.U.V.A., zweite, vermehrte und verbesserte Auflage, Wien, 1974.

17. Moore, M.L.: The Measurement of Joint Motion, Part I - Introductory Review of Literature, Phys. Ther. Rev., 29:195-205, May, 1949.

18. Moore, M.L.: The Measurement of Joint Motion, Part II - The Technic of Goniometry, Phys. Ther. Rev., 29:256-264, June, 1949.

19. Moore, M.L.: The Measurement of Joint Motion, Part III - Reliability of Goniometry, Phys. Ther. Rev., 29:303-307, July, 1949.

20. Müller, M.E.: Untersuchung der unteren Extremität Unter Besonderer Berücksichtigung der Prüfung der Gelenkbeweglichkeit mit der Nulldurchgangsmethode, Praxis: 59:526-530. 1970.

21. Müller, M.E., Boitzy, A.: La Cotation Chifree de Mobilite Articulaire. Medecine et Hygiene, Berne, 1970.

22. Nomina Anatomica (4th Ed.): Excerpta Medica, Amsterdam/Oxford, 1977.

23. Orthopedic Equipment Co.: O.E.C. International Standard S.F.T.R. Goniometer, Catalog Number 238, O.E.C., Bourbon, Indiana, 1962.

24. Orthopedic Equipment Co.: International Standard S.F.T.R. Pocket Goniometer, Catalog Number 240, O.E.C., Bourbon, Indiana, 1970.

25. Rippstein, J.: Neue Messgeräte für Klinik und Praxis in der Traumatologie, Hefte zur Unfallheilkunde, Heft 148, 3. Deutsch-Osterreichisch-Schweizerische Unfalltagung in Wien; Oktober, 1979; Springer-Verlag Berlin Heidelberg, 1980.

26. Rippstein, J.: Le Plurimetre-V64, Ann. Kinesietherapie, t. 10, No. -12, pp. 37-45, 1983.

27. Rippstein, J.: Nouvelle Technique Pour La Mensuration Des Mouvements Articulaires, Ortho-Scop, No. 11, pp. 23-32, 1984.

28. Rippstein, J.: Mess - Methodik für die Unfallmed. Begutachtung (Messbüchlein) von Hans Iselin, Basel; Schwabe & Co., Basel, 1932.

29. Rippstein, J.,: Poly - Goniometer, pp. 38-56, Teufel, Stuttgart, 1974.

30. Rippstein, J.: Das PLURIMETER MESSYSTEM 75 Jahre Klinik Balgrist, pp. 31-38 Verlag G. Thieme, Stuttgart, 1989.

31. Rowe, C.: Joint Motion of Measuring and Recording. American Academy of Orthopedic Surgeons, 1965.

32. Russe, O.A., Gerhardt, J.J., Machacek, J., Popp, O.: Atlas Orthopaedischer Erkrankungen. An Atlas of Orthopedic Diseases. pp. 26-43 Verlag, Hans Huber, Bern, Stuttgart, 1964.

33. Russe, O.A., Gerhardt, J.J., King, P.S.: Atlas of Examination, Standard Measurements and Diagnosis in Orthopedics and Traumatology. pp. 46-151 Verlag, Hans Huber, Bern, Stuttgart, Wien, 1972.

34. Russe, O.A.: Gelenkmessung, Neutral-0-Methode, SFTR-Notierung. Allgemeine Unfallversicherungsanstalt, Wien, 1972.

35. Russe, O.A., Gerhardt, J.J., Russe, O.J.: Tshenbuch der Gelenkmessung, Neutral-0-Methode, SFTR-Notierung. Verlag, Hans Huber, Bern, Stuttgart, Wien, 1974.

36. Schlaaff, J.: Hilfsmittel zur Einheitsmessung von Gelenkausschlägen, Der Messfächer "Arthro" und der Fingerfächer nach Schlaaff, Medizinal-Markt No. 11, p.413, 1957.

37. S.U.V.A. (Schweizer Unfall Versicherungs Anstalt). Spezielle Orthopädische Untersuchung, 1972.

38. Personal Communications:

Blount, W.P., M.D.
Böhler, L., M.D.
Boynton, B.L., M.D.
Erlacher, P.H., M.D.
Fox, Th. A., M.D.
Heck, C.V., M.D.

Hendryson, I.E., M.D.
Kolis, J., M.D.
Machacek, J. M.D.
Moore, M.L.
Ormbeck, G., M.D.
Popp, O., M.D.

Rippstein, J., M.D.
Rogers, T.M., M.D.
Rowe, C.R., M.D.
Russe, O., M.D.
Schlaaff, J., M.D.
Sofield, J., M.D.

John J. Gerhardt M. D.
Associate Clinical Professor in Orthopedics and Rehabilitation

Diplomate American Board of Physical Medicine and Rehabilitation
Fellow American Academy of Physical Medicine and Rehabilitation
Affiliations:
1. N. W. Permanente P. C. Department of Physiatry
    Kaiser Sunnyside Medical Center
    Clackamas, Oregon
2. Oregon Health Sciences University
    Portland, Oregon
3. Shriners Hospital for Crippled Children
    Portland, Oregon
4. Veterans Administration Hospital
    Portland, Oregon

Address: P.O. Box 588, Clackamas, Oregon 97015 U.S.A.

Jules Rippstein M.D.
Orthopedic Surgeon

Address: CH-1093 La Conversion, Champs des Pierrettes 53, Switzerland

Marie L. Valleroy M.D.
Staff Physiatrist, Medical Illustrator

Diplomate American Board of Physical Medicine and Rehabilitation
Fellow American Academy of Physical Medicine and Rehabilitation
Affiliations:
1. Rehabilitation Institute of Oregon
2. Good Samaritan Hospital and Medical Center
    Portland, Oregon

Address: 1040 N. W. 22nd, Suite 530, Portland, Oregon 97210 U.S.A.

Brian W. Demings A.A.M.I., A.B.P.A.

Affiliations:
1. Shriners Hospital for Crippled Children
    Portland Unit, Portland, Oregon
2. Association of Medical Illustrators
3. Biological Photographic Association

Address: 3101 S. W. Sam Jackson Park Road, Portland, Oregon 97201 USA

John J. Gerhardt / Philip King / Joseph H. Zettl

Immediate and Early Prosthetic Management – Rehabilitation Aspects

Foreword by E. M. Burgess. 2nd Edition of «Amputations».
1986 305 pages, 514 figures, softcover Fr. 84.— / DM 98.— /
US-Dollar 38.00 / Canadian Dollar 54.00

In the search for optimal postsurgical management of patients undergoing emergency or elective amputation, the immediate postsurgical prosthetic fitting (IPPF) has emerged as the best guarantee for a complete recovery and functional outcome. Despite being misunderstood by some to be equivalent to immediate weight bearing, and claimed by others to inhibit wound healing, the IPPF method has proven to be an effectiv and safe approach to the rehabilitation of amputees, especially those of the evergrowing geriatric population. Contents:

- Introduction and Historical Development
- Advantages of the Method
- Indications and Contradindications
- Assessment of Circulation
- The team Preoperative Planning
- Surgery
- Prostheses
- Conclusions and Research Outlook

 Verlag Hans Huber
Bern Stuttgart Toronto

Walter Dick

Internal Fixation of Thoracic and Lumbar Spine Fractures

Foreword by Prof. E. Morscher, M. D. Translation by James Wilson-MacDonald, M. D. 1989, 131 pages, 125 figures, 15 tables, hardcover Fr. 98.— / DM 118.—

This book is a major contribution to the on-going discussion surrounding the surgical treatment of vertebral fractures, in particular of the thoracic and lumbar vertebrae.
The autor speaks from long experience at the University Orthopedic Clinic and the Swiss National Paraplegic Center in Basel, and illustrates the book generously. The result of his work has been the development of a completely new, very short stabilizing system for the spinal column that no longer depends biomechanically on multiple fixation, but is itself stable on all axes. This internal fixation system also has since been clinically tested. In this book the author reports on his experience with some 200 patients over a 4-year period. In addition to giving detailed descriptions of the operative techniques with a number of practical tips he also describes his own methods of bone transplantation.

Robert Schneider

Total Prosthetic Replacement of the Hip

A Biomechanical Concept and its Consequences. Foreword by M. E. Müller. 1989, 335 pages, 233 illustrations (whereof 46 in color), hardcover Fr. 254.— / DM 298.—

This book is not for neophytes. But for the practitioner interested in state-of-the art techniques for surgery of the hip, it offers a gold mine of suggestions and thoughtful guidance. The material here is based on the author's experience with over 3300 hip replacements over the last 20 years.

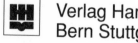
Verlag Hans Huber
Bern Stuttgart Toronto